D1175572

Manual of Clinical Dialysis

Second Edition

Manual of Clinical Dialysis

Second Edition

Suhail Ahmad

University of Washington, Scribner Kidney Center,
Northwest Kidney Centers, Seattle, Washington, USA

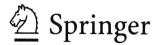 Springer

Suhail Ahmad, MD
Professor, Medicine
University of Washington
Scribner Kidney Center
Northwest Kidney Centers
Seattle, Washington
sahmad@u.washington.edu

ISBN: 978-0-387-09650-6   e-ISBN: 978-0-387-09651-3
DOI: 10.1007/978-0-387-09651-3

Library of Congress Control Number: 2008928866

Printed on acid-free paper

springer.com

Grateful thanks to my family, Vimli, Saba, and Zeba, and friends for their strong support and to Arlene for all of her help. This work is dedicated to my teachers, namely Dr. Scribner, and all of my patients.

Foreword (For First Edition)

As the next millennium begins, we hope that in the years ahead the need for dialysis will be decreased by better preventive care, especially the control of hypertension during the early stages of chronic renal disease. An increase in the number of donated kidneys and a decrease in their rejection rate also seems possible. In the meantime, it is our goal as dialysis professionals to do the very best job we can to make dialysis treatments as effective as possible in terms of patient survival and *rehabilitation.*

Despite the excellence of this manual, in terms of dialysis dose, one conclusion is inescapable: the current recommendation for dialysis dose, although recently revised upward, is still too low to support the well-being needed for rehabilitation. Indeed, at a urea reduction ratio of 65%, which is the current minimum set by Medicare, patients remain chronically uremic. The author does not say this, but if you read between the lines, he is trying to tell the reader that it is true. Furthermore, this dosage is based on observed (often malnourished) body weight, whereas it should be based on ideal body weight to reflect more accurately the needed dose.

Equally bad for patient well-being is the fact that there is no margin of safety built into this minimum. I believe a margin of safety is essential since the delivered dose is not checked with every dialysis; yet every aspect of dialysis procedures works against delivering the prescribed dialysis dose. For example, if adverse intradialytic events occur during a session, the time lost is seldom made up.

It is important to point out that the higher the weekly dose of dialysis the better. No adverse effects have been encountered no matter how high the dose. Pierratos has shown, with seven nights per week of home dialysis, a marked improvement in well-being, using a dose so large that phosphate had to be added to the dialysate.

Access to the circulation still is the "Achilles heel" of hemodialysis, and recirculation is a major cause of under-dialysis. The native Cimino fistula remains the gold standard. Vein grafts should never be used in patients in whom any natural vein is usable.

In the case of peritoneal dialysis, the danger of under-dialysis is ever present. Since the contribution by the native kidney in controlling uremia is more important in this group of patients, loss of residual renal function puts patients at risk for severe under-dialysis. In this group the close monitoring of the dose, including that supplied by residual renal function, is particularly critical to avoid adverse patient outcome.

The basic constraint that Dr. Ahmad has to live with in order to be realistic in his dosage recommendations is the "standard" $3^1/_2$ h, three times a week dialysis schedule. Both dialysis professionals and their patients must come to understand the basic fact that it is not possible, except in small patients, to give enough dialysis in $3^1/_2$ h, three times a week, to support rehabilitation. The current dismally low rehabilitation rate supports this contention. As suggested in the text, there are many ways to get beyond this session time constraint, and I hope these suggestions will increase interest in pursuing them according to the needs of the individual patient because under-dialysis is a major cause of failure to rehabilitate dialysis patients.

Of course, as soon as ways are found to break through this $3^1/_2$ h, three times a week session time barrier, other benefits begin to fall into place, such as correction of chronic acidosis and especially the ability to control blood pressure. It is my opinion, which is based on a huge amount of practical experience and published material, that antihypertensive medications are totally ineffective in controlling blood pressure in the dialysis population. In addition, their use increases the incidence of hypotensive episodes, especially during short dialyses. Indeed, antihypertensive medications must be discontinued before the patient's extracellular volume can be reduced to the level of dry weight. I define dry weight as that which reflects an extracellular volume small enough to render the dialysis patient normotensive and unable to tolerate antihypertensive medications. However, all this important information cannot be applied unless at least 12–15 h per week are devoted to being on dialysis.

Even if professional staff optimize every aspect of dialysis according to the guidelines in this manual, there still remains a key task. Staff must convince the patients of the vital importance to their well-being of receiving the highest possible dose of dialysis. Physicians in particular have proven to be poor advocates and teachers of this crucial objective. Patients must be made to understand that the higher the weekly dialysis dose, the better they will feel. Then it is up to the patients to decide whether it is a worthwhile trade off to spend extra time on dialysis in exchange for better sense of well-being, without which rehabilitation is very difficult if not impossible.

Seattle, Washington, USA   *Belding H. Scribner, MD*
July, 1999

Acknowledgements

Table 2.4 is adapted with permission from: ANSI/AAMI RD62: 2006 with permission of the Association for the Advancement of Medical Instrumentation, Inc. (C) 2006 AAMI www.aami.org. All rights reserved.

Figure 4.7 is adapted with permission from: Uldall R. Hemodialysis access. Part A: Temporary. In *Replacement of Renal Function by Dialysis, 4th Edition*. Edited by C Jacobs, CM Kjellstrand, KM Koch and JF Winchester. Dordrecht: Kluwer, 1996, pp. 277–293. © Kluwer.

Figure 5.6 is adapted with permission from: Golper TA, Wolfson M, Ahmad S et al. Multicenter trial of L-carnitine in maintenance hemodialysis patients. I. Carnitine concentrations and lipid effects. *Kidney Int* 1990, 38:904–911.

Figure 6.4 is adapted with permission from: 14. Daugirdas JT, Depner TA. A nomogram approach to hemodialysis urea modeling. *Am J Kidney Dis* 1994, 23:33–40.

Tables 7.2 and 7.8 are reproduced with permission from: Kaplan AA. Continuous arteriovenous hemofiltration and related therapies. In *Replacement of Renal Function by Dialysis. 4th Edition*. Edited by C Jacobs, CM Kjellstrand, KM Koch and JF Winchester. Dordrecht: Kluwer Academic Publishers, 1993:390–418. © Kluwer.

Figure 8.1 is adapted with permission from: Twardowski ZJ. Physiology of Peritoneal Dialysis. In *Clinical Dialysis, 3rd Edition*. Edited by AR Nissensson, RN Fine, and DE Gentile. Norwalk: Appleton and Lange,1995, pp. 322–342.

Figure 8.2 is reproduced with permission from: Nolph KD, Miller F, Rubin J et al. New directions in peritoneal dialysis concepts and applications. *Kidney Int* 1980, 18(Suppl 10):111–116.

Table 7.1 reproduced with permission from Mehta RL, McDonald BR, Aguilar MM, et al. Regional citrate anticoagulation for continuous arteriovenous hemodialysis in critically ill patients. Kidney Int 1990, 38:976–981

Tables 7.3 and 7.4 adapted with permission from Daugirdas JT, Blake PG, Ing TS: Handbook of Dialysis, 4th ed. Philadelphia, PA: Lippincott, William & Wilkins, 2007

Table 7.6 reproduced with permission from Swartz R, et al. Improving the delivery and continuous renal replacement therapy using regional citrate anticoagulation. Clin Nephrol 2004, 61:134–143

Table 9.5 is reproduced with permission from: Diaz-Buxo JA. Clinical use of peritoneal dialysis. In *ClinicalDialysis, 3rd Edition*. Edited by AR Nissenson, RN Fine and DE Gentile. Norwalk: Appleton & Lange,1995, pp. 376–425.

Figure 10.1 is reproduced with permission from: Diaz-Buxo JA. Chronic peritoneal dialysis prescription. In *Handbook of Dialysis, 2nd Edition*. Edited by JT Daugirdas and TS Ing. Philadelphia: Lippincott-Raven, 1993, pp. 310–327. © Lippincott, Williams & Wilkins.

Figure 10.2 is adapted with permission from: Diaz-Buxo JA. Clinical use of peritoneal dialysis. In *Clinical Dialysis, 2nd Edition*. Edited by AR Nissenson, RN Fine, and DE Gentile. Norwalk: Appleton & Lange, 1990, 13:256–300.

Figure 10.3 is adapted with permission from: Twardowski ZJ et al. Peritoneal equilibration test. *Perit Dial Bull* 1987, 7:138–140.

Table 11.5 is reproduced with permission from: Gokal R. Peritoneal infections, hernias and related complications. In *Replacement of Renal Function by Dialysis, 4th Edition*. Edited by C Jacobs, CM Kjellstrand, KM Kochand JF Winchester. Dordrecht: Kluwer, 1996, pp. 657–688. © Kluwer.

Table 11.6 is reproduced with permission from: Bargman JM. Noninfectious complications of peritoneal dialysis. In *The Textbook of Peritoneal Dialysis*. Edited by R Gokal and KD Nolph. Dordrecht: Kluwer, 1994:555–591. © Kluwer.

Figure 12.1 is reproduced with permission from: Lowrie EG, Lew LN. Death risk in hemodialysis patients: the predictive value of commonly measured variables and an evaluation of death rate differences between facilities. *Am J Kidney Dis* 1990, 5:458–482.

Table 12.3 is reproduced with permission from: Fouque D, Kopple JD. Malnutrition and dialysis. In *Replacement of Renal Function by Dialysis. 4th Edition*. Edited by C Jacobs, CM Kjellstrand, KM Koch and JF Winchester. Dordrecht: Kluwer, 1996:1271–1290. © Kluwer.

Figures 13.3 and 13.4 are reproduced with permission from: Charra B, Calemard E, Cuche M et al. Control of hypertension and prolonged survival on maintenance hemodialysis. *Nephrol* 1983, 33:96–102.

Figure 13.2 reproduced with permission from Eknoyan G, Beck GJ, Breyer JA et al. Design and preliminary results of the mortality and morbidity of hemodialysis (MMHD) pilot study [Abstract]. J Am Soc Nephrol 1994, 5:513.

Figure 13.9 is adapted with permission from: Buonchristiani U, Fagugli RM, Pinciaroli MR et al. Reversal of left ventricular hypertrophy in uremic patients by treatment of daily hemodialysis (dhd). *Contrib Nephrol* 1996, 119:152–156.

Table 13.3 is adapted with permission from: London G, Marchais S, Guerin AP. Blood pressure control in chronic hemodialysis patients. In *Replacement of Renal Function by Dialysis, 4th Edition*. Edited by C Jacobs, CM Kjellstrand, KM Koch and JF Winchester. Dordrecht: Kluwer, 1996:966–990. © Kluwer.

Figure 15.1 is reproduced with permission from: Rose BD, Rennke HG. Signs and symptoms of chronic renal failure. In *Renal Pathophysiology*. Edited

by BD Rose and HG Rennke. Baltimore: Williams & Wilkins, 1994:276–300.
© Lippincott, Williams & Wilkins.

Published by Science Press Ltd, 34–42 Cleveland Street, London W1P 6LB, UK.
© 1999 Science Press Ltd.

First published 1999. Reprinted 2000, 2003.

http://www.science-press.com/

British Library Cataloguing in Publication Data.

A catalogue record for this book is available from the British Library.

ISBN 1-85873-345-6

Project editor: Mark Knowles

Illustrator: Stuart Molloy

Typesetter: Simon Banister

Designer: Claire Huntley

Production: Adrienne Hanratty

Printed in Singapore by Stamford Press

Contents

Abbreviations

AII	Angiotensin II
AAMI	Association for the Advancement of Medical Instrumentation
ACE	Angiotensin-converting enzyme
ACT	Activated clotting time
AMAC	Arm muscle area circumference
AN6	Acrylonitrile-6
ARB	Angiotensin (II) receptor blockers
AV	Arteriovenous
AVP	Arginine-vasopressin
BIA	Bioelectric impedance analysis
BP	Blood pressure
BSA	Body surface area
BUN	Blood urea nitrogen
(i)Ca	(Ionized) calcium
CAAPD	Continuous automated ambulatory peritoneal dialysis
CAPD	Continuous ambulatory peritoneal dialysis
CAVH	Continuous arteriovenous hemofiltration
CAVHD	Continuous arteriovenous hemodiafiltration
CCB	Calcium channel blocker
CCPD	Continuous cycling peritoneal dialysis
CHF	(Slow and) continuous hemofiltration
CTS	Carpal tunnel syndrome
CVVH	Continuous venovenous hemofiltration
CVVHD	Continuous venovenous hemodiafiltration
DDS	Dialysis disequilibrium syndrome
DEXA	Dual-energy X-ray absorptiometry
DFO	Deferoxamine
DI	Dialysis index
DOQI	Dialysis Outcome Quality Initiative
DPI	Dietary protein intake
ECF	Extracellular fluid

ESRD	End-stage renal disease
Epo	Erythropoietin
Eto	Ethylene oxide
FBV	Fiber bundle volume
GFR	Glomerular filtration rate
GU	Glucose uptake
HCO_3	Hydrogen bicarbonate
Hct	Hematocrit
HD	Hemodialysis
HDF	Hemodiafiltration
HDL	High-density lipoprotein
HF	Hemofiltration
ICF	Intracellular fluid
IHF	Intermittent hemofiltration
IDPN	Intradialytic parenteral nutrition
IJ	Internal jugular
IPD	Intermittent peritoneal dialysis
IUF	Intermittent ultrafiltration
K_{urea}	Urea clearance
(e)Kt / V	(Equilibrated) dose of dialysis
KoA	Mass transfer coefficient
K_{ru}	Residual renal urea clearance
K_{uf}	Ultrafiltration coefficient
kd	Kilodalton
LDL	Low-density lipoprotein
LMWH	Low molecular weight heparin
LVH	Left ventricular hypertrophy
MAK	Mechanical artificial kidney
MCV	Mean corpuscular volume
MM	Middle molecule
MMHD	Morbidity in Maintenance Hemodialysis Study
NCDS	National Co-operative Dialysis Study
NIPD	Nocturnal intermittent peritoneal dialysis
NKF	National Kidney Foundation
NO	Nitric oxide
NTx	Cross-linked N-terminal telopeptide of type I collagen
PAN	Polyacrylonitrile
(n)PCR	(Normalized) protein catabolic rate
pClCr	Peritoneal creatinine clearance
pCl_{urea}	Peritoneal urea clearance
PD	Peritoneal dialysis
PET	Peritoneal equilibration test
PGI_2	Prostacyclin
PICP	Procollagen type I C-terminal peptide
pKt	Peritoneal urea clearance rate

PMMA	Polymethylmethacrylate
(n)PNA	(Normalized) protein equivalent of nitrogen appearance rate
PO_4	Phosphate
PTFE	Polytetrafluoroethylene
PTH	Parathyroid hormone
PTT	Prothrombin time
PTX	Parathyroidectomy
pre-BUN	Predialysis concentration of blood urea nitrogen
post-BUN	Postdialysis concentration of blood urea nitrogen
PS	Polysulfone
PV	Plasma volume
Qb	Blood flow rate
Qd	Dialysate flow rate
RBC	Red blood cell
rClCr	Renal creatinine clearance
rClU	Renal urea clearance
RO	Reverse osmosis
ROD	Renal osteodystrophy
RRT	Renal replacement therapy
SCUF	Slow and continuous UF
SGA	Subjective global assessment
SLED	Slow low efficiency dialysis
SM	Small molecule
SUF	Sequential ultrafiltration and dialysis
t	Time
TBW	Total body water
TIBC	Total iron-binding capacity
TMP	Transmembrane pressure
TPN	Total parenteral nutrition
TPD	Tidal peritoneal dialysis
TPR	Total peripheral resistance
TSFT	Triceps skin fold thickness
UF(R)	Ultrafiltration (rate)
UKM	Urea kinetic modeling
UNA	Urea/nitrogen appearance
URR	Urea reduction ratio
V	Volume of distribution of body fluid
VDR	Vitamin D receptors
V_{urea}	Volume of distribution of urea
WBC	White blood cell
W(p)ClCr	Weekly (peritoneal) creatinine clearance

Chapter 1
Brief History of Clinical Dialysis: The Seattle Experience

Although it was not until the 1960s that long-term dialysis in a clinical setting became a reality, dialysis as a treatment for renal failure had been the focus of interest for some time. By the end of the 1950s, Dr. B. H. Scribner had established an acute dialysis program at the University of Washington. In 1960, a uremic comatosed man who was thought to have acute renal failure was brought back to almost normal active life with intermittent hemodialysis. However, he was found to have chronic irreversible renal disease and had to be sent home to die; it became clear to the Seattle team that if long-term vascular access could be maintained, long-term dialysis would become a reality. This led to the development of the Scribner Shunt and the advent of chronic hemodialysis.

The Seattle team developed an entire program to care for a population of patients who had a chronic disease and who were being kept alive on a new form of treatment. New equipment and systems were developed and refined and solutions for unexpected problems had to be devised—specifically, treatment of hyperphosphatemia, renal osteodystrophy, and hypertension. To make the treatment more practical, by reducing the bulk of the dialysate through the use of concentrated dialysate, a proportioning system had to be developed and a substitute for bicarbonate was used to prevent the precipitation of calcium carbonate. This was achieved by using acetate. However, when acetate-related problems started to appear (due to the use of more efficient dialyzers, in the mid-1970s), a double proportioning system was developed to enable the use of bicarbonate again. As is often the case, the resolution of one problem often led to other unexpected difficulties. The commitment and ingenuity of the pioneers of dialysis treatment, however, meant that these hurdles were overcome and the success of dialysis as a treatment for end-stage renal disease (ESRD) was assured. Later in the 1980s, another Scribner fellow, Joseph Eschbach, developed and used recombinant erythropoietin, and anemia-related issues became history. The pioneering work continues today; the most recent modification in dialysate was the development of a citric acid-based acid concentrate for dialysate. This is proving to be more beneficial to the patients than the currently used acetic acid-based acid concentrate.

S. Ahmad, *Manual of Clinical Dialysis*, DOI 10.1007/978-0-387-09651-3_1,
© Springer Science+Business Media LLC 2009

The shortage of resources in the early days of dialysis necessitated the founding of a patient selection committee to decide which of the needy patients would be accepted into the program. This committee (thought by many to be the foundation for the development of medical ethics) forced several actions with far-reaching consequences, one of which was the development of home dialysis.

A young high-school student was found to have ESRD but was not accepted for dialysis by the patient selection committee. The team decided that home dialysis was a viable alternative if they could develop a smaller hemodialysis machine that could be used at home. The collaborative effort of Dr. Scribner's clinical team and the engineering team of Dr. Albert L. Babb succeeded in building a home hemodialysis machine in only 3 months. This home machine became the prototype of machines in use currently.

In early 1960s, Dr. Fred Boen joined the Seattle group and began treating a patient using peritoneal dialysis (PD), with a closed system containing 20-l (and later 40-l) bottles. Henry Tenckhoff, a research fellow with Dr. Boen, treated patients at home using Boen's repeated puncture technique. This technique, however, required aseptic access to the peritoneal cavity with a catheter each time dialysis was needed, and meant that Dr. Tenckhoff had to visit each patient's home at least three times a week to insert the access device. Eventually, Dr. Tenckhoff developed the indwelling peritoneal catheter and a sterile technique for its insertion, which made it possible to use the new form of dialysis on a larger scale.

A detailed analysis of the Seattle experience with intermittent PD (IPD) revealed the potential risk of under-dialysis and poor "technique survival rates" [1], suggesting that the dialysis dose needed to be increased. In 1965, Dr. Robert Popovich while in Seattle had become involved in the kinetics of the "middle molecule" across the peritoneal membrane before moving to Texas and becoming a pioneer of the continuous ambulatory PD (CAPD) technique. This continuous therapy improved the dialysis dose and made PD a viable technique of renal replacement therapy (RRT).

Encountering a patient who was dying of malnutrition due to bowel disease, Dr. Scribner saw an opportunity to apply the group's expertise in vascular access to another area of medicine. The development of Broviac (and later on Hickman) catheters and the "total parenteral nutrition" (TPN) program (operated by the nephrology team at the University of Washington) was a result of the vision and dedication of Dr. Scribner and his co-workers.

This very brief account of the Seattle experience shows that the commitment of Dr. Scribner, his team, their collaborators, and community members accomplished more than the development of a dialysis access device. Their efforts led to the development of systems for dialysis, central venous catheters, parenteral nutrition, long-term care of ESRD patients, community-based dialysis centers, home dialysis programs, an early concept of dialysis dose calculation, and continued technological improvement. The development of the dialysis program established nephrology as a subspecialty and has also had far-reaching implications in the fields of bowel disease, organ transplantation, oncology, and for all acutely ill patients. It is now difficult to imagine that less than 50 years ago, patients with ESRD had only one prognosis—death—and that patients with renal failure were connected to patients with liver failure so that each could be kept alive by the healthy organ of the other.

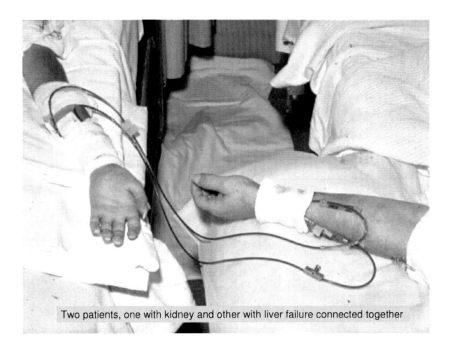

Two patients, one with kidney and other with liver failure connected together

1.1 Definition of Dialysis

In broad terms, the process of dialysis involves bidirectional movement of molecules across a semipermeable membrane. Clinically, this movement takes place in and out of blood, across a semipermeable membrane. If the blood is exposed to an artificial membrane outside of the body, the process is called hemodialysis (HD) or hemofiltration (HF). If the exchange of molecules occurs across the peritoneal membrane, the process is called peritoneal dialysis (PD).

1.2 Mechanisms Involved in Molecular Movement

The movement of molecules follows certain physiological and physicochemical principles that are outlined below (see Fig. 1.1a).

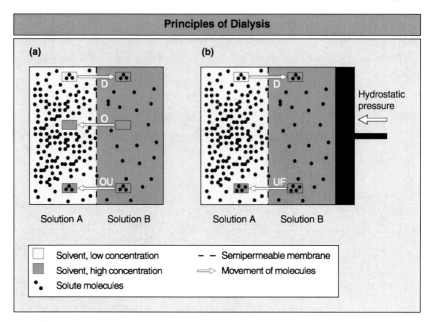

Fig. 1.1 a Diffusion, osmosis, and osmotic ultrafiltration by osmotic pressure. **b** Hydrostatic ultrafiltration. *D* diffusion, *O* osmosis, *OU* osmotic ultrafiltration, *UF* ultrafiltration by hydrostatic pressure, *C* convection

1.2.1 Diffusion

If two solutions of different concentrations are separated by a semipermeable membrane, solute will move from the side of higher to the side of lower solute concentration. This process of solute movement on a concentration gradient is called *diffusion* and is caused by the random movement of the solute molecules striking and moving across the membrane. Several factors influence this random movement and thus the rate of diffusion. The transport of any solute or solvent molecule is dependent on the *physical size of the molecule* relative to the size of the pores in the membrane. Any molecules larger than the pores of the membrane cannot pass through. Similarly, the *electrical charge* and the *shape* of the molecule also determine the rate of transport across the membrane. If the membrane has a negative charge, particles with a like charge will have limited transport as compared with those with a positive or a neutral charge.

1.2.2 Ultrafiltration

A solvent such as water can be forced across a semipermeable membrane on a pressure gradient, from higher to lower pressures (see Fig. 1.1). The pressure could be a result of osmotic force (see below) or of mechanical hydrostatic pressure. The solvent carries with it the dissolved solute molecules small enough to pass through the membrane pores (see below). This movement of molecules across a semipermeable membrane, caused by a pressure difference, is called *ultrafiltration* (UF). If the pressure is hydrostatic, the process is called "hydrostatic UF." Conversely, the UF caused by osmotic pressure is called "osmotic UF."

1.2.3 Osmosis

As solute concentration increases, solvent concentration correspondingly decreases and vice versa. If a semipermeable membrane separates solutions of different concentrations, solvent along with dissolved small solutes will flow from the side with the higher solvent concentration to the side with the lower solvent concentration. This process is called *osmosis* (see Fig. 1.1).

1.2.4 Convection

As solvent molecules move on a pressure gradient, the dissolved solute molecules are dragged along (solvent drag); this process of solute movement is called *convection*. The ease with which the solute is dragged along is determined by the size of the solute molecule relative to the size of the membrane pores. Smaller solutes are transported easily and the entire solution can sieve across the membrane without any change in concentration. In contrast, larger solutes move more slowly and the rate of convective transport is slower. Thus, the convective transport of a solute depends on the porosity of the membrane. This porosity, known as the "sieving coefficient of the membrane," can be calculated by dividing the concentration of solute on side A by the concentration on side B.

1.3 Clearance

In a clinical setting, the removal of a solute is measured in terms of clearance, the term being defined as the volume of blood or plasma from which the solute is completely removed in unit time. Let us assume that the blood urea concentration across a hemodialyzer drops from 100 mg/dl at the inlet to 10 mg/dl at the outlet. This 90% decline represents the diffusion of urea from blood into the dialysate and depends largely on the concentration gradient between these fluids. However, the magnitude of the "cleaning" of blood also depends on blood flow rates (Qb). Thus, in the above example, a blood flow rate of 100 ml/min means that 90 ml of the blood was cleared of urea. However, for a blood flow of 200 ml/min, 180 ml of blood is cleared of urea each minute (see the example below for a more accurate calculation). Clearance measures the magnitude of blood cleaning, independent of the concentration of the solute entering the dialyzer.

1.3.1 Blood vs Plasma Clearance

During transit across the dialyzer, most solutes are removed from plasma water (about 93% of blood volume, depending on plasma protein concentration). If the solute is not in the blood cells or if the movement of solute out of these cells is slow, the clearance of the solute decreases as the hematocrit increases (since the plasma volume decreases). Urea is often used as a solute to measure dialysis efficiency (it is present in plasma water as well as in erythrocytes), and the flux of urea across the erythrocyte membrane is reasonably fast. This means that urea is cleared from whole blood during dialysis and is not affected greatly by the hematocrit. The following example clarifies these concepts:

Example

Qb = 200 ml/min, hematocrit = 35%

Plasma flow rate = 200ml/min × (1 − 0.35) = 130ml/min

Plasma water flow rate = 130 ml/min × 0.93 (93% of plasma is water) = 121 ml/min

Erythrocyte flow rate = 200 ml/min − 130 ml/min = 70 ml/min

Erythrocyte water flow rate = 70 ml/min × 0.80 (about 80% of erythrocyte volume is water [containing diffusible urea]) = 56 ml/min

Thus, the whole blood water flow rate effective for urea clearance = 121 ml/min + 56 ml/min = 177 ml/min

If the blood water concentration of urea = 100 mg/dl at dialyzer inlet and 10 mg/dl at outlet, the urea clearance of whole blood = 177 ml/min × {1 − [(10 mg/dl)/ (100 mg/dl)]} = 159 ml/min

This means that 159 ml of blood is cleared of urea each minute.

1.3.2 Clinical Factors Influencing Dialysis Urea Clearance

The three major determinants of urea clearance during hemodialysis are:

Blood flow rate (Qb)

Dialysate flow rate (Qd)

Membrane (dialyzer/peritoneal membrane) efficiency

Reference

1. Ahmad S, Gallagher N, Shen F. Intermittent peritoneal dialysis: status reassessed. *Trans Am Soc Artif Intern Organs* 1979, 25:86–89.

Chapter 2
Hemodialysis Technique

As discussed in the previous chapter, the clearance of a solute is dependent on the Qb, Qd, and membrane efficiency. The dialyzer membranes have different pore sizes that are variably distributed, larger pores being fewer than smaller pores. Small solutes like urea can be transported through all pore sizes whereas the larger molecules such as vitamin B12 or beta-2-microglobulin can only pass through the larger pores. Thus the clearance of the larger solutes, unlike urea, is more influenced by the membrane and less by Qb and Qd.

2.1 Blood Flow Rate

Because clearance is calculated using Qb, it would be understandable to mistakenly assume that the relationship between urea clearance and Qb is linear. However, although urea clearance increases steadily as Qb is increased from zero, at faster flow rates, the dialyzer is unable to continue to transport urea with the same efficiency and the urea concentration at the dialyzer outlet increases. In other words, the urea removed as a percentage of urea inflow into the dialyzer decreases and (as clearance is Qb multiplied by the fractional decline in urea) the clearance curve plateaus (see Fig. 2.1).

2.2 Dialysate Flow Rate

An increase in Qd generally increases the urea clearance. This effect is negligible, however, as long as Qd is 150–250 ml/min faster than Qb. With high-efficiency dialyzers, there is little (<10%) increase in urea clearance if Qd is increased from 500 ml/min to 800 ml/min, provided that Qb remains 350 ml/min.

S. Ahmad, *Manual of Clinical Dialysis*, DOI 10.1007/978-0-387-09651-3_2,
© Springer Science+Business Media LLC 2009

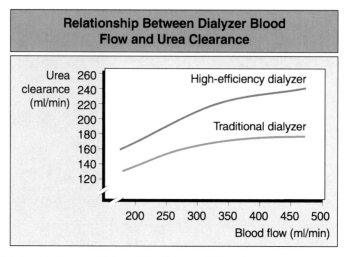

Fig. 2.1 Relationship Between Dialyzer Blood Flow and Urea Clearance

2.3 Dialyzer Efficiency and Mass Transfer Area Coefficient (KoA)

Dialyzer efficiency is measured in terms of clearance at a given Qb and Qd. Usually, these values are measured for urea and other solutes at a Qb of 200 ml/min and a Qd of 500 ml/min. Another measure of dialyzer efficiency is solvent removal in terms of the ultrafiltration coefficient (K_{uf}). However, dialyzer efficiency is more accurately measured as the mass transfer coefficient (KoA). The KoA of a solute is defined as the maximum (theoretical) ability of a membrane to allow the transfer of a solute through its pores when Qb and Qd are unlimited. Thus, KoA is the clearance of a solute when dialysate and blood flow are not the limiting factors. The higher the value of KoA, the more permeable the membrane for that solute. Thus, the higher KoA of a dialyzer for a solute, the more that solute would be cleared, and this value is proportional to the surface area and porosity of a membrane. However, if the surface area becomes too large, the relationship will not remain linear (this will be further discussed later).

2.4 Different Hemodialysis Techniques

2.4.1 Traditional Hemodialysis

In traditional hemodialysis, blood flows on one side and the dialysate on the other side of a dialyzer membrane (see Fig. 2.2). To maximize solute movement, the blood and dialysate flow in opposite directions (counter current flow). In this technique,

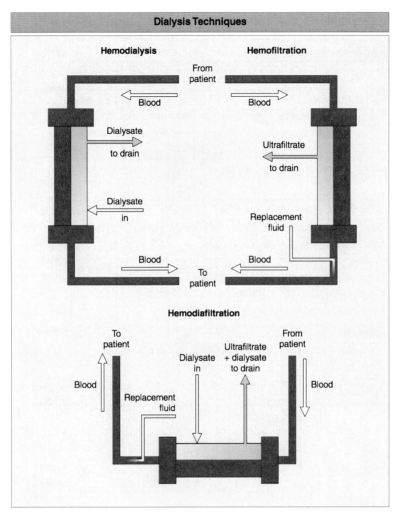

Fig. 2.2 Replacement fluid can be added to the circuit either before (pre-dilution) or after (post-dilution) the dialyzer/filter

diffusion is the predominant method of solute clearance. There is a very small amount of hydrostatic UF to remove the excess fluid volume (usually 2–3 l) gained between dialysis sessions, contributing a small solute clearance by convection.

2.4.2 Hemofiltration

The technique of hemofiltration (HF) uses a large quantity of hydrostatic UF. Plasma ultrafiltrate is replaced with plasma-like electrolyte solution. Solute removal is achieved by convection (solvent drag), and volume control by the difference between the volume removed and the volume replaced (see Fig. 2.2). This technique can be intermittent (IHF) or slow and continuous (CHF). CHF is used in acute renal failure and uses an arterial catheter to remove blood from the patient and a venous catheter to return the blood. This technique is called continuous arteriovenous hemofiltration (CAVH). The same technique, using only a dual-lumen venous catheter, is called continuous venovenous hemofiltration (CVVH).

2.4.3 Hemodiafiltration

In order to improve solute clearance, hemofiltration (convective transport) may be combined with diffusive transport by allowing dialysate to flow on the ultrafiltrate side. Intermittent use of this technique is called hemodiafiltration (HDF) (see Fig. 2.2), while continuous use (commonly used in acute renal failure) is called continuous arteriovenous hemodiafiltration (CAVHD) or continuous venovenous hemodiafiltration (CVVHD), depending on the location of the catheter(s).

2.4.4 Slow Low Efficiency Dialysis (SLED)

Slower removal of solutes is better tolerated than rapid removal. Thus, in an acutely ill patient, sometimes the slow removal is achieved by reducing the dialysate flow to 300 ml/min or lower with blood flow not exceeding 200 ml/min, and the treatment time is prolonged to 8–24 h. This technique, slow low efficiency dialysis (SLED), is better tolerated with less hemodynamic instability.

2.4.5 Ultrafiltration

If volume removal alone is needed, it can be achieved by intermittent UF (IUF) or slow and continuous UF (SCUF), without replacement of ultrafiltrate.

2.5 Hemodialysis Setup

Hemodialysis apparatus can be divided in two major components (see Fig. 2.3):

Blood circuit
Dialysate circuit

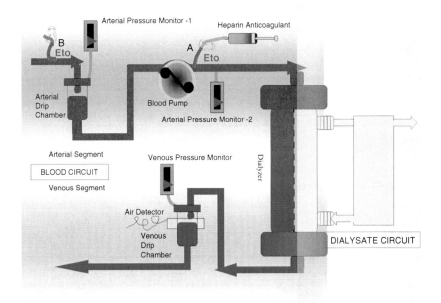

Fig. 2.3 Hemodialysis Setup

2.5.1 Blood Circuit

The blood circuit comprises:

Tubing set with ports, drip chambers, and an access device
Blood pump
Hemodialyzer

2.5.1.1 Tubing Set

Blood is drawn from the patient into the blood tubing, either through a central venous catheter or through a needle inserted into the patient's vascular access (fistula or graft). Blood tubing can be divided into two major segments. The segment that carries blood from the patient to the hemodialyzer is traditionally called the "arterial segment," while the segment that carries blood from the dialyzer back to the patient is called the "venous segment." Usually, each of these segments has a drip chamber into which blood flows and any air rises to the top. Blood drains from the drip chamber into the blood tube, continuing its course toward the dialyzer from the arterial and to the patient from the venous drip chamber. Pressure in these segments is monitored (arterial pressure monitor 1 in arterial drip chamber located before the blood pump and venous pressure monitor in the venous drip chamber), and if it goes beyond the set ranges, the alarm sounds and the blood pump stops. The venous drip chamber also has a level and air detector. If the blood level drops below the detector level because of too much air, an air alarm sounds, the pump stops, and the tubing segment below the drip chamber is clamped to prevent any air being introduced into the patient. Some systems have an additional arterial pressure monitor between the blood pump and the dialyzer (arterial pressure monitor 2) that enables the reading of pressure between the pump and the dialyzer. The pressure in the arterial segment before the pump (monitor 1) is negative and after the pump (monitor 2) is positive, reflecting the resistance caused by the dialyzer. Pressure in the venous segment is positive, reflecting the resistance caused by the vascular access. The drop in pressure between post pump pressure and venous pressure represents the effect of ultrafiltration. For the calculation of transmembrane pressure (TMP), either the average of the two pressures (if post pump arterial pressure is measured) or the venous pressure is used. The TMP is the pressure on the blood side of the dialyzer membrane minus the pressure on the dialysate side. The blood tubing is usually sterilized using ethylene oxide (Eto), thus, the blood tubing needs to be thoroughly rinsed prior to connecting the tubing to the patient.

> Caveat: Pre-setup rinsing of the blood segment must remove all ethylene oxide (Eto), failure to do so often causes an allergic reaction in the patient during the treatment. When this happens despite a thorough rinse, the allergic reaction is usually caused by inappropriate rinsing procedure and/or a poorly constructed tubing set. As shown in Fig. 2.3, during the rinse, Eto backed up in the heparin line (Eto shown as purple, A&B); if the heparin line is not flushed before connecting to the patient, the heparin pump will inject Eto into the patient first, causing an allergic reaction (Fig. 2.3A). Figure 2.3B shows that a poorly constructed clamp left a small segment where the Eto can collect during the rinsing process, and the patient eventually may be exposed to this Eto during the treatment, evoking a reaction. To avoid this, the clamps on the side branches should be good quality and close to the main tubing segment. The procedure should ensure flushing of the heparin and other side branches during the rinse cycle.

2.5.1.2 Blood Pump

The most common type of blood pump is the roller design. Rotating rollers compress the pump segment of the tubing and sweep the blood forward. The speed of rotation determines Qb. The usual Qbs range from 200 to 500 ml/min in adults (median rate about 350 ml/min). If the pump is set at a certain rate but access is unable to provide blood at that rate, the pressure in the arterial chamber 1 drops below the set range and the alarm stops dialysis. Similarly, any excessive resistance to blood being returned to the patient increases pressure in the venous drip chamber and the system will stop if the set range is exceeded. There are two access-related reasons for insufficient blood flow—that the arterial segment is not receiving the desired blood flow or that the venous side cannot return the flow back to the patient. The former means that the pump is causing too much negative pressure. This pressure limit is usually set at −200 mmHg, with any drop below this limit sounding the alarm. Problems with the return of blood cause the pressure in the venous drip chamber to increase and a pressure greater than 200 mmHg is usually considered unsafe.

   The blood pump is a "demand driven" pump; thus, the blood pump rotation (flow rate) is set at a fixed rate and the pump "demands" blood at this rate. The design of the pump is inflexible, leading to frequent alarm interruptions. The other common problem with the blood pump is the trauma the rollers cause to the pump segment of the blood tubing (spalling), limiting the tubing's useful life [1]. The pump segment tubing material is silicone rubber and the rest of the blood tubing is usually made of polyvinyl chloride. The diameter of the pump tubing segment determines the "stroke volume" of blood per sweep. This requires that the rollers completely occlude the tubing segment, incomplete occlusion would reduce the stroke volume and Qb. At a very high pump speed, often the arterial pressure becomes too negative and tubing may partially collapse, again reducing the stroke volume and Qb. To get the reliable Qb, the pump needs to be frequently checked and calibrated.

2.5.1.3 Hemodialyzer

The dialyzer is the site of the movement of molecules (dialysis process) and is the critical part of the dialysis apparatus. It contains a semipermeable membrane, through one side of which flows blood and the other side dialysate. This membrane consists of either thousands of capillary fibers (hollow fiber dialyzers) or of a sheet that is arranged in parallel plates (parallel plate dialyzers). The hollow fiber design is the version used most frequently (see Fig. 2.4). The major components of this are:

Blood ports—carry blood into (arterial port) and out of (venous port) the dialyzer
Headers—from the blood port, the blood enters the arterial header space and dialyzed blood enters the venous header space (before entering the venous blood port)

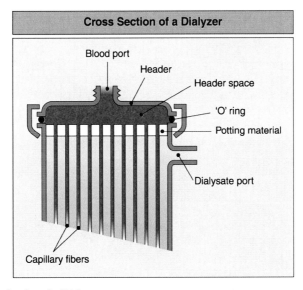

Fig. 2.4 Cross Section of a Dialyzer

Potting material—the hollow capillary fibers are anchored to the dialyzer casing
with a potting material, separating the blood from the dialysate compartment

Space between header and fibers—this critical space is where clotting most often
occurs

Capillary fibers—about 10,000 capillary fibers made of permeable material are
contained within the dialyzer casing. The blood flows inside the fibers and the
dialysate flows on the outside

Dialysate ports—there are two ports on the side of the casing, one for dialysate
inflow and one for the outflow

Space between ports and potting material—this space is critical because dialysate
flow (and thus clearance) in this space is relatively poor

Dialyzer Characteristics

Selection of a dialyzer is based on material and performance characteristics:
  Membrane: The material that constitutes the membrane can be divided into four
broad groups:

 (i) Cellulose membrane: Early material derived from plant polysaccharide was
     called cellophane. Later, other forms of cellulosic materials (based on the
     manufacturing process) were used; these included cuprophan (cuprammonium
     cellulose), saponified cellulose ester, and regenerated cellulose. The cellulosic
     membranes were widely used and are less expensive than the other membrane
     materials but cause more immunoactivation. Their use in the USA over recent
     years has declined because of being less bio-compatible.
 (ii) Substituted cellulose membrane: The cellulose membranes described above
     contain free hydroxyl groups that are thought to activate complements when
     exposed to blood. In an attempt to reduce this, free hydroxyl groups have been
     bonded to materials like acetate to form substituted cellulose membranes such
     as cellulose acetate, diacetate, and triacetate. These are thought to be more bio-
     compatible.
(iii) Mixed cellulosic–synthetic membrane: During the manufacturing process, a
     tertiary amine compound is added to the cellulose thus the membrane sur-
     face becomes more biocompatible. These membranes are called Hemophan
     (Cellosyn).
(iv) Synthetic membrane: Several synthetic membranes are currently in use. These
     differ from cellulosic membrane in several aspects. The synthetic membranes
     are generally more biocompatible, have higher hydraulic permeability, and are
     more expensive. Some of these membranes also adsorb plasma proteins, im-
     munoglobulins, and complements. Common synthetic membranes materials
     include polysulfone (PS), polyacrylonitrile (PAN), polycarbonate, polymethyl-
     methacrylate (PMMA), and polyamide.

  Biocompatibility of the membrane: The dialyzer membranes cause activation of
blood cells, complement blood cells, and complement cascade. This is thought to

occur mostly by free hydroxyl moieties present on the surface of cellulosic membranes. The activated cells produce cytokines and lead to various clinical sequelae and dialytic reactions. Antioxidants are also produced during dialysis and new dialyzers are being produced in which the membrane is coated with antioxidant materials such as vitamin E. The use of these dialyzers has been reported to be associated with less production of oxidants. The biocompatibility is attributed to the membrane material, with cellulosic membranes being the least biocompatible, synthetic membranes the most biocompatible, and others in between. The potting materials as well as the middle layer (the layer between the two skins of the membrane) can also cause bio-incompatibility.

- Dialyzer performance: Dialyzer performance is judged by solute clearance and UF characteristics:

(i) Solute clearance: The solute removal characteristic of a dialyzer is one of the key measures of its performance. It is reported in terms of clearance of solutes such as urea, creatinine, phosphate (PO_4), uric acid, beta-2-microglobulin, and vitamin B_{12}. Clearance depends on the thickness and surface area of the membrane and on the density, characteristics, and size of the pores.

Urea clearance is the most commonly used measure, since it is used in the calculation of the dose of dialysis. The clearance data provided by the manufacturer usually comes from in vitro experiments using water and is always higher than the blood clearance obtained in vivo. Therefore, the manufacturer's in vitro data must not be used to determine the dialysis prescription using urea kinetics. Generally, creatinine clearance is 70–95% of urea clearance. PO_4 and uric acid clearances are not always reported but can be useful in treating markedly elevated PO_4 or uric acid levels (e.g., those encountered with tumor lysis syndrome and acute renal failure). However, PO_4 is an intracellular ion and, using a dialyzer with a high PO_4 clearance, the plasma value can fall quickly without a major impact on total body removal of this ion. Vitamin B_{12} (with a molecular weight of 1355) has lower clearance and helps in defining the permeability of the dialyzer for larger (middle) molecules. Recently, beta-2-microglobulin clearance has also been used as a method of assessing membrane characteristics, particularly the flux of the membrane.

(ii) UF characteristic: The UF characteristic of a dialyzer is measured as the K_{uf}, the volume of plasma water removed per hour per mmHg of TMP, and is reported in terms of the ultrafiltration rate (ml/h/mmHg). Thus, the UF rate (UFR) can be accurately calculated for each treatment from the K_{uf} of the dialyzer and TMP during the procedure.

Example

A dialyzer with a K_{uf} of 4 ml/h/mmHg is used for a treatment. The prepump arterial pressure is −100, the post-pump arterial pressure is not measured, the venous pressure is 100 mmHg, and the patient needs to lose 2.7 kg during a

3-h run. What should be the dialysate pressure to achieve the above UF goal if no UF modeling is used?

$TMP = P_b - P_d$ and $UFR = TMP \times K_{uf}$; $UFR = 2,700\,ml/3$ h, or $900\,ml/h$
where P_b is the pressure on the blood side and P_d is the pressure on the dialysate side of the membrane
$900\,ml/h = TMP \times 4\,ml/h/mmHg$; or $TMP = 900\,ml/h \div 4\,ml/h$ or $225\,mmHg$
$225\,mmHg = P_b - P_d$, or $225 = 100 - P_d$; or $P_d = -125\,mmHg$, or the dialysate side would have to supplement the blood side pressure by having a negative pressure
If a dialyzer with a K_{uf} of 15 is used and rest of the variables remain unchanged, the 100 mmHg venous pressure would cause more UF than desired, in this case, the P_d would be positive to slow down the UFR by countering the P_b
$TMP = 60$ and $P_d = 40$ (P_b remains 100).

From the above example, it is clear that dialyzers with a high K_{uf} can cause excessive UF and need fine balancing of pressure from the dialysate side in order to prevent over ultrafiltration. Thus the dialyzers with a K_{uf} of >8 ml/h/mmHg should only be used with machines with volumetric control ability. In dialyzers with a very high K_{uf} (such as 100 ml/h/mmHg), a large pressure drop occurs along the length of the capillary fiber and often a back-leak of dialysate occurs or even a small leak in the membrane can cause infusion of dialysate from the venous end of the fibers into the blood. For this reason, very porous dialyzers may be safe only with ultrapure dialysate.

Surface area and porosity of the membrane: Dialyzer clearance is dependent on the porosity of the dialyzer and the total surface area of the dialyzer membrane. The surface area of most dialyzer membranes ranges from 0.8 to 2.1 m². For the less biocompatible membranes such as cuprophan, the larger the surface area, the more potential there is for immunoactivation (see below).

Priming volume: Priming volume is the volume of the blood compartment of the dialyzer and is therefore equal to the volume of blood that will fill this compartment. For dialyzers used with adults, this volume ranges from 50 to 150 ml.

Membrane thickness: Usually, thin membranes are more permeable than thicker membranes. However, thinner membranes cannot withstand as high a TMP as thicker membranes.

In addition to dialyzer performance characteristics, the dialyzer sterilization technique may be of importance. The most common method of sterilization is with Eto. Removal of Eto prior to use of the dialyzer is very important because some patients experience a severe anaphylactic reaction to small amounts of Eto, which is difficult to remove from the potting material without thorough rinsing. In Eto-sensitive patients, only dialyzers sterilized by alternative methods (e.g., gamma radiation or steam autoclaving) should be used. Because of the risk of severe reaction to Eto, this method is becoming less commonly used and gamma radiation and steam sterilization are becoming more popular.

High-Efficiency High-Flux Dialyzers

Dialyzers that are more efficient and contain high flux membranes have become very popular during the last two decades. It is worthwhile to clarify the various membrane characteristics because confusion regarding the definitions and terminology is prevalent. Flux: The term flux defines the ability to ultrafilter plasma water, or the K_{uf} of a membrane. Thus, a membrane with K_{uf} of <10 ml/h/mmHg is called a low-flux membrane and a membrane with >20 ml/h/mmHg is called a high-flux membrane. Efficiency: Efficiency denotes the solute removal by diffusion based on the KoA of urea; membranes with a KoA urea of <500 ml/min are called low-efficiency membranes and those with >600 ml/min are called high-efficiency membranes. Generally, the high-flux dialyzers also have high-efficiency membranes and vice versa. However, theoretically, the two could be very different (Fig. 2.5).

Mass transfer area coefficient (KoA): As discussed in Chapter 1, the KoA is the clearance of a solute at infinite Qb and Qd, usually expressed in terms of urea clearance or KoA$_{urea}$. This theoretical value can be calculated from clearance and blood and dialysate flows:

$$KoA = (Qb \times Qd)/(Qb - Qd) \times \ln[(1 - Ks/Qb) \div (1 - Ks/Qd)],$$

where Ks = the dialyzer clearance of a solute such as urea. Thus, the KoA value is more affected by clearance than Qb or Qd.

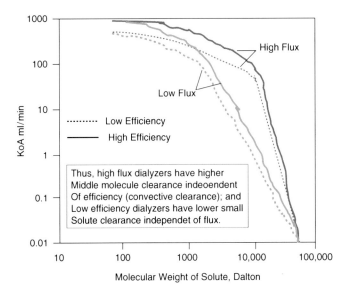

Fig. 2.5 Clearances of different size solutes by low and high efficiency and low and high flux dialyzers

Reuse of Dialyzers

Traditionally, dialyzers have always been reprocessed and reused—mainly for convenience and to save time. With the popularity of the more expensive high-efficiency dialyzers, cost saving has become the major factor for reuse. However, recently, the interest has shifted from reuse to no reuse, because of the concern about the process and its effect on the treatment and patient. Although there is no clear evidence of reuse having any adverse effect on patients or treatment, some reports even have cited the possible benefit of reuse. With no reuse, the cost of dialysis supplies increases, and the impact on the environment by increasing the amount of contaminated waste is of major concern.

The reuse technique involves rinsing with clean water and/or cleaning agents such as sodium hypochlorite (bleach), hydrogen peroxide, or peracetic acid. After thorough cleaning, the dialyzer is sterilized; formaldehyde is the most common agent used but glutaraldehyde has also been used for this purpose, and there has been interest in using heat. Before the dialyzer is used again, several safety checks are mandatory:

Dialyzers are tested chemically to ensure that no sterilizing agent remains.
Membrane patency is checked by the use of a pressure test.

Dialyzer efficacy is tested to ensure that enough membrane surface is still available for dialysis. This is done by measuring the fiber bundle volume (FBV). If the FBV is >80–85% of the baseline value, the dialyzer is deemed to have an adequate number of patent fibers. Any dialyzer with a lower value should be discarded.

2.5.2 Dialysate Circuit

The major components of the dialysate circuit (Fig. 2.6) are:

Dialysate
Dialysate delivery system

2.5.2.1 Dialysate

These days, bicarbonate dialysates are almost exclusively used for dialysis. Concentrated dialysate that is proportioned by mixing with treated water in the machines is the most common form. However, mixing of concentrated $NaHCO_3$ and $CaCl_2$ leads to the precipitation of $CaCO_3$.

$$CaCl_2 + NaHCO_3 \rightarrow Ca(HCO_3)_2 + NaCl \rightarrow CaCO_3 + H_2O + CO_2$$

The precipitation is avoided by separating the concentrated $NaHCO_3$ (B-concentrate) from the rest of the constituents of the dialysate (A-concentrate). To further reduce the risk of $CaCO_3$ formation, an acid is added to the A-concentrate, this keeps the pH of the final dialysate below 7.4 after the proportioning and mixing of the A- and B-concentrates. The lower pH drives the equation to the left, resulting in more soluble calcium chloride and calcium bicarbonate instead of less soluble calcium carbonate formation. Based on the acidifying agent, two types of A-concentrates are available:

Acetate-containing acid concentrate (acetate dialysate): The acid concentrate contains acetic acid, usually 4 mEq/l (in liquid concentrate) or 8 mEq/l (in powdered concentrate, Granuflo® Fresenius) in the final dialysate.

Citrate-containing acid concentrate (citrate dialysate): The predominant acid is citric acid, usually 2.4 mEq/l, with 0.3 mEq/l acetic acid (Citrasate®, Advanced Renal Technologies). The composition of the rest of the constituents is identical in the two forms of dialysate.

Clinical effects: The presence of citric acid has been reported to have some beneficial effects, mostly related to its anticoagulant properties (Table 2.1). During the recent years, there have been concerns about acetate causing activation of cells and inflammatory markers. There is a lot of interest in further reducing or removing acetate from the dialysate.

Liquid versus dry concentrate: Both acetate- and citrate-containing concentrates are available in either dry form or liquid form. The dry concentrate is dissolved in appropriate volume of treated water before connecting it the machine. Examples of dry forms are Granuflo® (8 mEq/l acetate) by Fresenius, and DRYalysate® (2.4 mEq/l citrate) by Advanced Renal Technologies. Examples of liquid formulations are Naturalyte® and Citrasate®, by Fresenius and Advanced Renal Technologies, respectively.

Table 2.1 The clinical effects of the two currently used acid concentrates

Type of dialysate	Disadvantages	Advantages
Acetate-containing bicarbonate dialysate	Intradialytic complications, Activation of cells Activation of inflammatory proteins	—
Citrate-containing bicarbonate dialysate	Decrease in Ca and Mg	Reduced clotting: • Increase in the dose of dialysis • Heparin-free acute/chronic dialysis • Reduced heparin chronic dialysis • Increase in reuse of dialyzer

The B-concentrate is usually 25 times concentrated and the A-concentrate either 35 or 45 times concentrated.

Bicarbonate concentrate: Bicarbonate is available in powder form. The powder is either mixed manually with appropriate volume of water prior to connecting to the machine, or the powder comes filled in a cartridge and is attached to the machine. With the cartridge form, the water is delivered to the cartridge and the concentrated solution is used directly from the cartridge by the machine.

Lactate-containing dialysate: In a small number of home dialysis patients using frequent and slower rate dialysis, the NxStage machine uses a dialysate that contains lactate in place of bicarbonate as a basic anion.

Thus, currently used dialysates contain bicarbonate as the predominant basic anion (used for the vast majority of patients) or lactate (used for only a small number of patients).

2.5.2.2 Dialysate Delivery System

The dialysate delivery system blends and provides dialysate to the dialyzer, monitors dialysate quality, and controls and monitors UF from the patient. It can be divided into four major components:

Water preparation system: Treated (purified) water (see Section 2.5.2.4) is delivered to the machine, where it is heated to an appropriate temperature (34–39°C) by a heater (see Fig. 2.6) and deaerated (usually by subjecting the heated water to a negative pressure, using a pump). Water is then delivered to the proportioning system.

Proportioning system: There are different types of proportioning systems based on whether dialysate, water, or both are metered. Simply stated, the proportioning system takes appropriate volumes (based on how concentrated the concentrate is) of parts A and B of the concentrate and mixes them with the appropriate volume of (in the appropriate ratio) treated water to form the final A and B dialysates, the final mixing of the two diluted parts A and B makes the final dialysate; the composition is shown in Table 2.2. The final dialysate is then checked for proper mixing (proportioning) by measuring the conductance of electricity through the final dialysate. The rate of flow of an electric current through any solution is proportional to the concentration of electrolytes present in the solution, thus, distilled water is a very poor conductor of electricity, and the salt solution is a good conductor. Thus, from the rate of electrical conductance, the concentration of salt in the solution can be verified. Roughly, the conductance is about 1/10th of the sodium concentration, thus a dialysate of 135 mEq/l sodium concentration should have a conductivity value of 13.5 ms/s. If the conductivity of the dialysate is in the acceptable range, the dialysate is allowed to proceed to the dialyzer. If the conductivity is out of range, the dialysate is diverted to the bypass loop. The temperature of the dialysate is also monitored prior to its passage through the dialyzer, if the temperature is out of range, the dialysate is diverted to bypass. It is important to have separate and independent sensors monitoring and controlling the proportioning units.

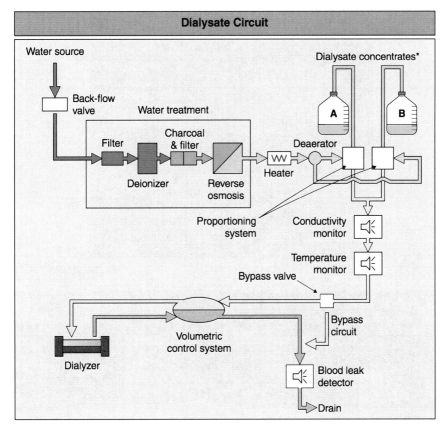

Fig. 2.6 Dialysis circuit

Volumetric-controlled machines: These machines have two integral parts to ensure accurate ultrafiltration, (1) the balancing chamber and (2) the UF controller (Fig. 2.7).

1. Balancing chamber: The risk of over-ultrafiltration because of the use of permeable dialyzers required the development of a machine that could accurately track the ultrafiltration and control the rate. This was achieved by ensuring that dialysate inflow into and outflow out of the dialyzer were same. The "balancing" of the two flows is most commonly achieved by allowing the inflow and outflow into a rigid chamber and keeping the two volumes separated by a diaphragm that deflects an equal distance from the middle. This balancing chamber concept works by inflowing a fixed volume into the chamber, and the fixed deflection of the diaphragm pushes an equal volume out of the chamber. The interplay of the four sets of one-way valves ensures that an equal volume of dialysate goes into and comes out of the dialyzer. Two sets of these balancing chambers acting in alternate cycles achieve a more continuous flow of the dialysate.

Table 2.2 Ranges of dialysate components. Citrate dialysate has 2.4 mEq/L citrate and 0.3 mEq/L acetate

Composition of Dialysate (mEq/l)	
Sodium	135 – 145
Potassium	0 – 4
Calcium	2.5 – 3.5
Magnesium	0.5 – 1.5
Chloride	98 – 112
Acetate /Citrate	4 – 10 / 2.4
Glucose	0 – 200 mg/dl
Bicarbonate	35 – 40

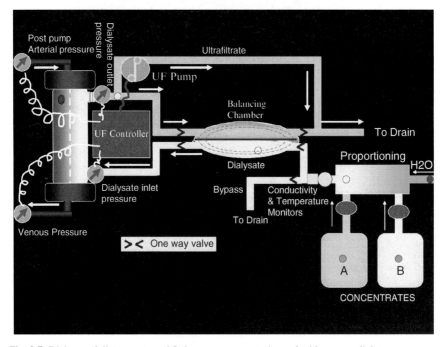

Fig. 2.7 Dialysate delivery system. *Only one concentrate is used with acetate dialysate

2. UF controller: A separate line branches out of the dialysate outflow line, the flow in this line is controlled by a UF pump. The pump in turn is controlled by a central computer unit that gets information from the dialyzer inlet and outlet pressures for both blood and dialysate; the unit also gets information about the

required rate and net volume of UF fed into the machine prior to the treatment. This computer unit then controls the UF rate by controlling the UF pump.

Monitors and detectors: For safety, several monitors and detectors are used in the dialysate delivery system:

(i) Conductivity monitor: As discussed earlier, the appropriate mixing of concentrate with water is monitored by conductivity. Because this monitor essentially checks the electrolyte concentrations in the final dialysate, any malfunction that is accompanied by abnormal proportioning can be potentially fatal for the patient. Any deviation from the narrow set range leads to the sounding of an alarm and the interruption of dialysis.

(ii) Temperature monitor: Patients need to be dialyzed with dialysate at 36–42°C. Dialysis at $<36°C$ is associated with the patient feeling cold and uncomfortable, and a dialysate temperature of $>42°C$ is associated with severe hemolysis and cardiopulmonary arrest. The dialysate temperature is monitored and a thermostat controls the water heater. Any increase in temperature beyond the set range triggers an alarm and dialysis is stopped (usual safe range set between 35–39 C).

(iii) Blood leak detector: Blood leak sensors are placed on the dialysate outflow line. These are usually flow-through photo-optical or blue frequency spectrum sensors.

(iv) pH sensors: Some machines have a pH electrode as part of the proportioning system. These are generally used to prevent any mistake in connecting the appropriate concentrates to the machine (e.g., B concentrate not being connected).

(v) Arterial and venous pressure monitors: Both arterial and venous drip chambers are connected to a pressure sensor through a filter. The pressure ranges are set in the safe range to monitor the blood delivery to and from the system. The prepump arterial pressure would usually be a negative number representing the demand by the pump. Generally, the safe lower limit of the arterial pressure is no lower than -100 mmHg. The venous pressure is generally kept below 200 mmHg.

(vi) Air detector: An air detector is located on the venous drip chamber. If too much air collects, an alarm sounds, the pump stops, and a blood line below the drip chamber is clamped to prevent an accidental infusion of air.

2.5.2.3 Dialysis Water

Drinking water contains chemical, microbiological, and other contaminants. A healthy adult drinks about 10–12 l of water per week, this water goes across a selective barrier of the gastrointestinal tract, and excess chemicals are removed by the healthy kidney. In contrast, during dialysis, a dialysis patient is exposed to more than 350 l of water weekly, the water passes through the nonselective dialyzer membrane, and there is no kidney to maintain the normal balance of chemicals. Moreover, the highly permeable high-flux membrane used today increases the risk of

Table 2.3 Toxic effects of water contaminants documented in HD patients

Toxic Effects of Water Contaminants Documented In HD Patients	
Contaminants	**Toxic Effects**
Aluminum	Encephalopathy, Bone Dis. Anemia
Calcium/Mg	Nausea, Vomiting, Weakness, Headache, HTN, Malaise, Cardiac Prob.
Copper	Hemolysis, Fever, Headache, Hepatitis
Chloramines	Hemolysis, Anemia, Methemoglobinemia
Fluoride	Bone Disease, Osteomalacia, Arrhythmia
Nitrate	Cyanosis, MetHb, Hypotension, Nausea
Sodium	HTN, Pulm.Edema, Headache, Thirst, Confusion, Seizure, Coma
Sulfate	Nausea, Vomiting, Acidosis
Zinc	Anemia, Nausea, Vomiting, Fever
Microbial Cont.	Chills, Fever, Septicemia, Liver Injury
Pyrogen	Pyrogenic Shock,

contaminants passing through the membrane and into the blood. Table 2.3 gives the commonly present contaminants and medical syndrome caused by these in dialysis patients. Some common contaminants have been shown to be injurious to patients. Contaminants include aluminum (causing bone and brain problems and anemia), copper (causing hemolytic anemia and febrile reactions), and chloramine (causing hemolytic anemia). If the large quantities of salt and electrolytes that are normally present in the water are allowed to remain, higher concentrations of these occur in the final dialysate. The Association for the Advancement of Medical Instrumentation (AAMI) has recommended minimum standards for the water used in dialysis (see Table 2.4) [2].

Thus, the water for dialysis must be purified of these contaminants prior to its use by the proportioning system of the dialysis machine.

2.5.2.4 Water Treatment System

Two major types of water purification systems are in common use: (1) reverse osmosis (R/O) and (2) deionizer (D/I). However, to protect and prolong the lives of R/O membrane or the D/I resins, water goes through several steps of "pretreatment" (Figs. 2.8 and 2.9).

Pretreatment system: The first component of the pretreatment system is a *sediment filter* that removes sediments such as silt, rust, and clay as water percolates through the filter. Next, there is a water *softener* that is filled with resin charged with NaCl; as water passes around these resin beads, the Ca and Mg in the water are exchanged with NaCl, thus, water coming out has less Ca and Mg. The softner is periodically recharged by flushing it with brine. The water next is passed through a set of *activated charcoal columns*. Some organic contaminants and especially the chlo-

Table 2.4 AAMI standard of water quality for dialysis

Substance	Maximum allowable concentration (mg/l)
Aluminum	0.01
Chloramines	0.1
Copper	0.1
Fluoride	0.2
Nitrate	2.0
Sulfate	100.0
Zinc	0.1
Arsenic	0.005
Barium	0.1
Cadmium	0.001
Chromium	0.014
Lead	0.005
Mercury	0.0002
Selenium	0.09
Silver	0.005
Calcium	2.0 (0.1 mEq/L)
Magnesium	4.0* (0.3 mEq/L)
Potassium	8.0* (0.2 mEq/L)
Sodium	70.0* (3.0 mEq/L)
Antimony	0.006
Free Chlorine	0.50
Thallium	0.002

*Maximum allowable error (adapted with permission from [2])

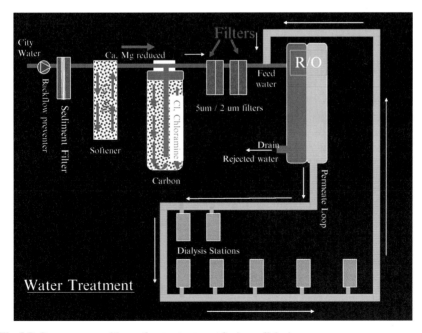

Fig. 2.8 Components and loop of water treatment for hemodialysis

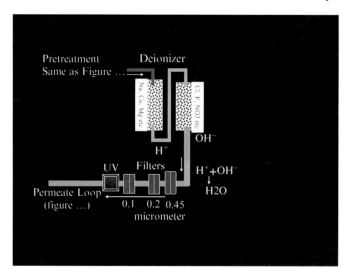

Fig. 2.9 Deionizer as the water purification method and associated components

rine and chloramines are adsorbed on the charcoal surface and removed from the water. This is important because chloramines can damage the R/O membranes and are not effectively removed by the D/I. Exhaustion of the charcoal column has led to several significant incidences of chloramine toxicity. It is, therefore, required that treated water is checked for chloramines at least three times a day to ensure proper functioning of the charcoal columns. Sets of several gradually decreasing sizes of *filters* (from 5 to 2 μm) are placed to remove smaller particles. The pretreated water is then passed through the final water treatment system, either R/O or D/I.

Reverse osmosis system (R/O): Membranes with very small holes are arranged in a cartridge either in the form of a parallel plate or capillary fibers. The holes are so small that they only allow water molecules to pass through, retaining anything larger, including sodium and urea. The pretreated water is forced through these holes by a pump that generates enough pressure to squeeze water molecules against higher osmolar pressure, thus, the name, reverse osmosis. The membrane separates the pure water or permeate from the "rejected" water, the pure water is allowed to circulate through the dialysis unit to be used for the dialysate proportioning; the rejected water is drained out. The R/O membranes are made from either cellulosic or synthetic materials. Cellulosic membranes are prone to be damaged by bacteria, whereas the synthetic membranes (polyamide, polysulfones, etc.) are more vulnerable to chemicals such as chloramines and chlorine. The efficacy of the membrane is continuously monitored by measuring the resistance to electrical current through the product (permeate) and feed water. A membrane that rejects >85% of conductant water is considered to be functioning well, if this rejection rate goes below 85%, the membrane needs to be changed. The rejection ratio $= (1 - $ [conductivity permeate/conductivity feed water]) $\times 100$. Deionization (D/I): Removal of inorganic ions by exchanging the inorganic ions with H^+ and OH^- ions is the process of D/I. The most common type is a mixed-bed D/I that consists of resins fixed with H^+ (cation) and other resins coated with OH^- ions (anion). As water with dissolved inorganic ions percolates first through the cation exchange resin, the dissolved cations (Na, Ca, Mg, etc.) are exchanged for H^+. Water then passes through the anion exchange resins and anions (Cl, Fl, NO_3, etc.) are exchanged with OH^-, H^+, and OH^-, then forming pure water that, after going through submicron filters and often ultraviolet light, is permitted to loop around the unit. The product water coming out of D/I is monitored by checking the resistivity, which should be greater than $1\,m\Omega/cm$ to be acceptable.

Most of the major catastrophies afflicting groups of patients have been caused by improperly treated water delivering contaminants to the blood. Thus, it is mandatory to use an effective water treatment system and to continuously monitor the quality of the water. Moreover, the increased use of highly permeable high-flux dialyzers increases the potential for the transfer of contaminants into the blood, thus, the water needs to be further purified. Some units use a tight membrane filter (dialyzer); the dialysate passes across this first dialyzer prior to its delivery to the patient dialyzer. This "ultrapure" dialysate further protects the patient.

References

1. Kim WG, Yoon CJ. Roller pump induced tubing wear of polyvinylchloride and silicone rubber tubing: phase contrast and scanning electron microscopic studies. *Artif Organs* 1998, 22:892–897.
2. ANSI/AAMI RD62: 2006 with permission of the Association for the Advancement of Medical Instrumentation, Inc. (C) 2006 AAMI www.aami.org. All rights reserved.

Chapter 3
Anticoagulation

Contact with a foreign surface leads to clotting of blood, because of the activation of intrinsic pathways and platelets. Clotting of the extracorporeal system stops the dialysis system, thus, the prevention of clotting is necessary for the dialysis to proceed. However, the partial clotting of dialyzer fibers or, more importantly, of the pores of the membrane, reduces the effective surface area, thus, reducing the efficacy of the treatment. The partial clotting of the pores of the membrane is one of the most under appreciated limitations of the treatment. The loss of the dialytic efficacy, particularly for the larger molecules, often goes unrecognized and inadequate dialysis in those patients who clot easily is very common. In one study when patients with lower Kt/V urea (K = dialyzer urea clearance, t = duration of dialysis, and V = volume of distribution of urea) were dialyzed against citrate-containing dialysate, the Kt/V urea increased significantly [1]. In another study [2], the Kt/V urea was significantly lower (Fig. 3.1) in those patients who had a limited number of reuses of dialyzer (most likely from loss of fiber bundle volume from clotting) than those with a higher number of reuses. With citrate dialysate, the number of reuses and Kt/V urea increased in the first group. These data point to the need for effective anticoagulation during the treatment. Further, the activation of the clotting cascade is known to produce proinflammatory proteins that, in turn, activate the inflammatory cascades; inflammation is commonly reported in dialysis patients. Unfortunately, dialysis patients are also at increased risk of bleeding due to platelet dysfunction, at the same time clotting of the extracorporeal system and of the vascular access is a common occurrence. These factors pose a major challenge to the proper management of dialysis patients. The other complicating factor is the differing sensitivity of patients (and sometimes the same patient at different times) to the most commonly used anticoagulant, heparin. Anticoagulation methods are described below (Fig. 3.2).

S. Ahmad, *Manual of Clinical Dialysis*, DOI 10.1007/978-0-387-09651-3_3,

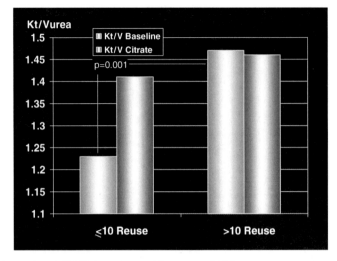

Fig. 3.1 Comparison of Kt/V in patients with lower and higher reuse on regular dialysate and citrate dialysate. (From Reference 2)

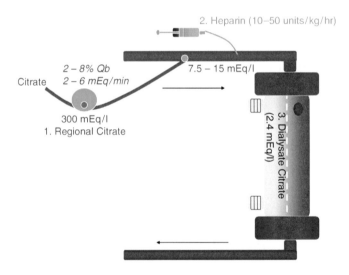

Three Common methods of anticoagulation

Fig. 3.2 Three common methods of anticoagulation during hemodialysis

3.1 Heparin Anticoagulation

The most common anticoagulant for dialysis continues to be heparin. Unfractionated heparin is a highly charged linear glycosaminoglycan (GAG) made up of repeating disaccharide units (typically 2–9 units), alternating amino sugar (glucosamine) and uronic acid residues. Heparin is largely metabolized by the liver and no dose adjustment in renal failure is needed. Heparin works by activating antithrombin and binding with thrombin and with factor Xa, thus, these important clotting cascade steps. Heparin anticoagulation leads to systemic anticoagulation of the patient thus increasing the risk of bleeding.

There are two main techniques of heparinization.

3.1.1 Systemic Standard Heparinization

The technique of systemic standard heparinization is most commonly used in stable chronic dialysis patients and initially a heparin bolus (about 2,000–3,500 U) is given, usually through the venous line of the dialysis access, to increase the baseline activated clotting time (ACT) to 200–250 s (normal range, 90–140 s). This bolus dose may be followed by continuous infusion of heparin (500–2,000 U/h) to maintain the ACT in the therapeutic range of two times baseline ACT. To prevent excessive bleeding, heparin must be discontinued 30–60 min before the termination of treatment. Some centers use a single bolus dose of heparin at the start of treatment, dose in excess of 5,000 U, and then 1,000-U boluses as needed. The latter method usually uses more heparin than the former. Unfortunately, in the USA, most centers have stopped monitoring ACT because of increased oversight requirements and expenses involved with the cost and maintenance of the machines. The efficacy of heparinization is judged by the inspection of the dialyzer and drip chambers at the termination of dialysis. With the decline in the reuse of dialyzer, unfortunately, the fiber bundle volume loss or decreased reuse as a measure of increased clotting is not available to judge the anticoagulation efficacy. More vigilance to prevent excessive clotting is needed.

3.1.2 Low-Dose Heparinization

If risk of bleeding is high, a more stringent heparin protocol is used in those patients at risk of bleeding—the target ACT in this situation being 150–200 s 1.25 times baseline. In general, a dose of 5–10 U/kg is administered, followed by either no heparin or a very slow infusion of 250–500 U/h. If ACT declines or if clotting is suspected, small bolus doses of heparin (e.g., 500 U) are administered in place of a continuous infusion.

3.1.3 Low Molecular Weight Heparin

Low molecular weight heparin (LMWH) is composed of smaller fractions of the heparin molecule (4–6 kDa). In contrast to unfractionated heparin, the LMWH does not bind thrombin but activates antithrombin and binds factor Xa. LMWH is administered as a single bolus at the start of dialysis and has been used safely in dialysis patients. Some of the claimed potential advantages (such as reduced risk of bleeding and beneficial effect on plasma lipids compared with heparin) have, however, not been proven and one study reported no significant benefit over citrate anticoagulation [3]. Because LMWH fractions are generally more expensive than heparin, it may only be useful if regular heparin or citrate cannot be used. The efficacy is measured by anti-Xa activity, which is not widely available. The dose is expressed as anti-Xa units (Institute Choay units) and the usual per treatment dose is 125–250 anti-Xa units/kg, with the lower dose (125 anti-Xa units/kg) used if there is risk of bleeding. Because of the expense, it is not widely used in the USA.

3.2 Problems with Heparin Anticoagulation

Heparin is an effective and inexpensive method of controlling coagulation, however, it has several major drawbacks (Table 3.1). The risk of excessive bleeding is its major limitation, under these condition, its use is limited. Thus, in the presence of active bleeding, presurgery, postsurgery, in major trauma, and in the presence of serositis, such as pericarditis, heparin cannot be used. *Heparin-induced thrombocytopenia* (HIT) seems to be increasingly diagnosed and, in the presence of heparin antibody, heparin use is contraindicated. LMWH also must not be used because the risk of cross reactivity is very high. *Hypertriglyceridemia and low HDL levels* have been reported with unfractionated heparin but not with LMWH, however, this has been disputed recently. *Hyperkalemia* caused by the suppression of aldosterone synthesis has been reported to improve slightly with the use of LMWH instead of unfractionated heparin. Other less common adverse events are listed in Table 3.1, however, recently, there have been more troubling reports about the *proinflammatory effects* of both unfractionated and LMW heparin compared with citrate anticoagulation, thus, this topic needs more attention. The outbreaks of infection caused by a contaminated heparin-filled syringe led to the recall of these syringes by the US

Table 3.1 Complications of heparin anticoagulation and some common alternatives

Complications	Alternatives
Bleeding risk, active bleeding	No heparin, low-dose heparin, citrate
Heparin-induced thrombocytopenia (HIT)	No heparin, citrate, heparinoids, thrombin inhibitors
Lipid disorders	Alternative agents
Osteoporosis	Not studied well
Pruritus	Alternative agents
Hyperkalemia	LMWH, alternative agents
Hair loss	Alternative agents
Induction of inflammation	Citrate

LMWH Low molecular weight heparin

Food and Drug Administration (FDA). Improperly manufactured heparin causing widespread fatalities have underlined the need for improved quality standards.

3.3 Alternatives to Heparin

Several alternatives to heparin anticoagulation have been used; all have some limitations in terms of expense, complexity, or length and irreversibility of the anticoagulation. Citrated dialysate has recently emerged as the least expensive and simplest alternative, although it is not universally effective.

3.3.1 Citrate Anticoagulation

Citrate is one of the best and longest used alternatives to heparin [4]. Citrate prevents clotting by binding with the calcium necessary for the clotting cascade. This type of anticoagulation is only effective as long as there is no calcium. The systemic circulation has enough calcium, and, once in the systemic circulation, the calcium citrate uncomplexes, the citrate is metabolized through Kreb's cycle, and the calcium is added to the calcium pool. The net result is that the citrate anticoagulates only the extracorporeal system, thus, there is no risk of increased bleeding. Two major methods of citrate anticoagulation are in common use.

3.3.1.1 Citrate Dialysate (Local Citrate) Anticoagulation

As discussed in Chapter 2, a new dialysate that contains 2.4 mEq/l of citrate in the final dialysate (Citrasate™ and DRYalysate™, Advanced Renal Technologies, Kirkland, WA, USA) appears to bind with calcium locally at the level of dialyzer membrane thus preventing the clotting of dialyzer capillary fibers and its pores. This novel method to use citrate in the dialysate has been successfully and safely used during the last 8 years in the USA. The use of new dialysate has been reported be associated with a significant increase in the delivered dose of dialysis without any other change in dialysis treatment variables. The authors have proposed that the presence of citrate in the dialysate keeps the dialyzer fibers and pores open, thus, increasing solute transport [6].

The evidence of this comes from several studies and wide use of citrate dialysate without heparin in both chronic and acute dialysis. Several studies have shown significant increase in dialysis dose associated with citrate dialysate, with the authors suggesting that the reduction in clotting at the local dialyzer level was responsible for this increase. Similarly, successful completion of dialysis with a significant reduction of heparin or heparin-free dialysis with citrate dialysate has also been reported; again, supporting the view that the small amount of citrate is effective in preventing clotting of the dialyzer. Advantages to this technique include its simplicity, just switch the acid concentrate, its low cost, and virtually no side effects of citrate even with long treatments of 20 h and in patients with multi-organ failure, including liver failure. There is no risk of bleeding, whether used in conjunction with heparin or heparin free, the heparin-free citrate dialysis has been successfully used intra-operatively during liver transplantation.

3.3.1.2 Regional Citrate Anticoagulation

Traditional method: Citrate is infused into the early arterial segment of the blood tubing, calcium is removed from the dialysate, and calcium is infused into the venous segment prior to returning the blood to the patient. Thus, the blood in the extracorporeal system is anticoagulated. Trisodium citrate solution (102 mmol/l) is infused at 2–6% of the blood flow rate (the rate is higher for the first few minutes of treatment and then it is decreased). Because of the potential for citrate toxicity (cardiac arrhythmia), a 4% citrate solution is now used in place of tri-sodium citrate. Infusion of calcium into the venous line restores the ionized calcium level before the blood is returned to the patient. This extracorporeal anticoagulation reduces the risk of bleeding. It is important to remember that the blood being returned to a patient should not be calcium free, since this can cause potentially fatal cardiac arrhythmias, especially if central venous catheters are used for dialysis access. For this reason, infusion of calcium should commence as soon as citrate infusion is started. A calcium chloride solution (made as a 3–5% solution and infused at a rate of 0.5 ml/min) can be infused into the venous tubing segment close to the patient.

Modified citrate anticoagulation: In an attempt to simplify the technique, citrate anticoagulation with a calcium-containing dialysate and without calcium infusion has been successfully used [5]. This simplifies the citrate anticoagulation procedure considerably, and although serum calcium needs to be monitored carefully, with proper attention and adjustment of calcium level, this method can be used without significant problems.

Citrate anticoagulation reduces the risk of bleeding and keeps the dialysis system free of clots. However, it has several disadvantages: it is more expensive than heparin, it has been associated with more fluctuations in serum calcium levels, and it can cause hypernatremia and alkalosis (Table 3.2). To avoid the latter two complications, the citrate solution should always be made in aqueous dextrose solution, and the dialysate bicarbonate concentration should be reduced to about 25 mEq/l.

3.3.1.3 Heparinoids

Heparinoids are mixture of heparin, dermatan, and chondroitin sulfates (e.g., Danaproid). These mostly block factor X activity and are renally excreted, thus, in renal failure, the half-life is prolonged. Danaproid can cross react with heparin antibody and should be used with caution.

Table 3.2 Comparison of three methods of anticoagulation

Issues	Heparin	Citrate dialysate (local)	Regional citrate
Cost	Least expensive	Relatively inexpensive	Most expensive
Anticoagulation efficacy	Very effective	Modestly effective	Very effective
Complexity	Requires pump or bolus, relatively simple	Very simple, just connect dialysate to machine	Very complex, monitoring of calcium required
Risk	Significant, bleeding and Table 3.1	Minimal (none reported)	Significant: hypernatremia, hypocalcemia, alkalosis, arrhythmia

3.3.1.4 Direct Thrombin Inhibitors

Direct thrombin inhibitors act by directly inhibiting thrombin thus blocking the terminal step in the clotting cascade. Argatroban is synthetic molecule that is metabolized in the liver and cannot be safely used in liver failure. Argatroban is usually administered as an initial bolus of 250μg/kg followed by infusion at a rate of 2μg/kg/min. Recombinant hirudin also inhibits both thrombin-induced and platelet-induced clotting but, unlike heparin, it does not cause platelet aggregation. Recombinant hirudin is administered as a single bolus at the start of dialysis. The prolonged half-life of hirudin in dialysis patients increases the risk of bleeding. Hirudin is also more expensive than heparin.

3.3.1.5 Prostacyclin and other Prostanoids

Prostacyclin and other prostanoids are potent platelet inhibitors. Prostacyclin has a very short half-life and has been used as a constant infusion of about 4 ng/kg/min. However, the expense and the incidence of side effects (including vasodilation and hypotension) limit its use.

3.4 No Anticoagulation

In patients at high risk of bleeding complications (particularly in acute cases), dialysis can often be successfully carried out without any anticoagulation, and several different approaches to this have been used. In one method, the dialyzer and tubing set are presoaked with 2,000–7,000 U of heparin for >30 min. It is important to rinse all heparin out before connecting the patient to the machine. Alternatively, periodic (every 30 min or so) rinsing of the blood circuit with saline minimizes the risk of clotting. Often both of these methods are used. In the majority of hospitalized patients, dialysis can be performed safely without anticoagulation, the only drawback being that the process is labor intensive.

Use of erythropoietin (Epo) to prevent anemia seems to be associated with increased clotting and, as such, requires better anticoagulation. With the popularity of high-flux and high-speed dialysis, it is important that appropriate attention to anticoagulation be paid, to avoid under dialysis (due to clotting of fibers) or access thrombosis.

References

1. Kossmann RJ, Gonzales A, Callan R, Ahmad S: Citrate Dialysate Decreases Aluminum Burden in Hemodialysis Patients. ASN abstract, 2008.
2. Ahmad S, Callan R, Cole J, Blagg C: Increased Dialyzer Reuse with Citrate Dialysate. Hemodial Int 9:264–267, 2005.
3. Janssen MJ, Deegens JK, Kapinga TH et al. Citrate compared to low molecular weight heparin in chronic hemodialysis patients. *Kidney Int* 1996, 49:806–813.
4. Pinnick E, Wiegmann TE, Diederich DA. Regional anticoagulation for hemodialysis in the patients at high risk for bleeding. *N Engl J Med* 1983, 308:258–261.
5. VonBrecht JH, Flanigan MJ, Freeman RM et al. Regional anticoagulation—hemodialysis with hypertonic trisodium citrate. *Am J Kidney Dis* 1986, 8:196–201.
6. Ahmad S, Callan R, Cole JJ et al. Dialysate made from dry chemical using citric acid increases dialysis dose. *Am J Kidney Dis* 35(3):493–499, 2000.

Chapter 4
Vascular Access

A long-term, reliable, dependable, and safe method of repeatedly accessing patient's blood has been, and continues to be, one of the most difficult challenges for hemodialysis therapy. The Scribner shunt was a milestone, allowing the use of long-term hemodialysis for the first time, but problems with thrombosis and infection were common, and the shunt is no longer commonly used. However, access-related issues continue to be the Achilles heel of hemodialysis management, exacting significant cost, morbidity, and mortality. Current access techniques can be divided into permanent and temporary access.

4.1 Permanent Access

4.1.1 Preparation

Preparation for a permanent access, preferably a fistula, must begin as soon the patient is diagnosed with progressive chronic kidney disease. Initially the preparation involves the preservation of peripheral veins as a future site. The importance of this cannot be emphasized enough, because these literally are to be the lifeline of the patient. Thus, venipuncture should only use most distal small veins or, if larger veins have to be used, a very experienced person should use these to prevent permanent damage or clotting. Indwelling lines, such as a peripherally inserted central catheter (PICC), in the peripheral veins must be avoided at all cost. If it cannot be avoided, then it perhaps is better to use a PICC in the central veins for the minimal possible duration.

A complete history and physical examination prior to the referral to the surgeon avoids potential problems later. Venous study by duplex Doppler is usually sufficient to aid the surgeon in selecting the best site. In unclear cases, venography can be used, as long as the risk of contrast media on the renal function are seriously considered.

S. Ahmad, *Manual of Clinical Dialysis*, DOI 10.1007/978-0-387-09651-3_4,
© Springer Science+Business Media LLC 2009

The starting diameter of the target artery and vein are often used as predictor of successful arteriovenous (AV) access. There is controversy about the minimum diameter of the starting vessels for a successful outcome, however, arterial and venous diameters of smaller than 1.5 mm usually do not result in a successful fistula. Some think that the minimum acceptable diameter of a vein should be 2.5 mm for a useable fistula. *Venous and arterial dilation tests* have also been proposed to predict the outcome; thus while doing the Doppler study, the occlusion of a vein leading to a 50% increase in the internal diameter of the vein is considered a predictor of a good fistula.

4.1.1.1 Preferred Access Choice

It is quite clear that the AV fistula is by far the preferred vascular access and, in every patient, this must be considered first. Kidney Disease Outcomes Quality Initiative (KDOQI) guidelines (2006) suggest the following preferences in order:

 (i) A wrist (radial–cephalic) primary AV fistula
 (ii) An elbow (brachial–cephalic) primary AV fistula

If the above are not possible, then:

 (iii) A transposed brachial basilic vein fistula
 (iv) An AV graft using synthetic material (such as polytetrafluoroethylene [PTFE])

The long-term use of cuffed tunnel catheters must be discouraged, and they should be used only as a last resort.

4.1.2 Arteriovenous Fistula

In the mid-1960s, Drs. Cimino, Brescia, and coworkers described the AV fistula, created by subcutaneous anastomosis of the cephalic vein and radial artery. Over time, the venous segment (receiving a large flow of arterial blood under pressure) dilates and develops a thickened wall (arterializes). This segment can be accessed with dialysis needles, providing blood for dialysis. To date, the AV fistula is by far the best method of vascular access. Review of the literature by the DOQI group found that the AV fistula has the "longest life with least complications" and a "longer intervention-free life" than any other vascular access method [1]. Thus, the AV fistula is the current method of choice for access.

4.1.2.1 Technique

Under appropriate anesthesia, the artery and veins are exposed surgically, and the distal end are brought to close proximity and anastomosed. The vessels are joined

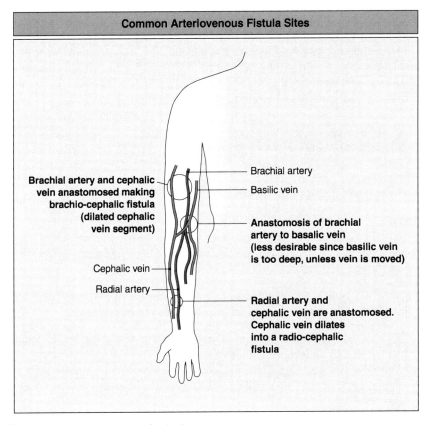

Fig. 4.1 Common arteriovenous fistula sites

side-to-side or the side of the artery is joined to the end of the vein (side-to-end). The most commonly used vessels are the radial artery and the cephalic vein (radio–cephalic fistula; see Fig. 4.1) [2].

With AV anastomosis, arterial pressure is transmitted to the vein, which dilates and thickens. The side-to-side technique may cause venous hypertension, leading to edema and discomfort in the hand. In the side-to-end technique, the distal part of the vein is tied and there is no venous hypertension. In contrast to the Scribner shunt (see below; Section 4.1.6.1), the artery remains patent and blood supply to parts distal to the anastomosis is open. However, anastomosis causes a low resistance flow from artery to vein, and blood may be diverted straight to the vein rather than through the distal capillaries; this may result in ischemic complications (steal syndrome).

In patients with forearm veins that fail to develop, an upper arm fistula may be used. The brachial artery and either the cephalic or the median cubital vein are joined side-to-side near the elbow to create a brachio–cephalic fistula (see Fig. 4.1). This type of fistula usually provides high flow, but the length of the usable venous segment is limited. Thus, this technique should be used only when the more distal radio–cephalic location is not available.

4.1.2.2 Fistula Use

Fistulae should not be used for at least 2 months after their creation, because use before the venous wall is mature can shorten its life. Some think that the longer the wait prior to use, the better the outcome of the fistula, so it is important that the need for dialysis is anticipated and a fistula is created months prior to its use.

4.1.2.3 Arteriovenous Fistula Complications

- Postoperative swelling, edema, and pain: These are common and tend to improve within a few days. Raising the arm usually helps to alleviate these symptoms.

(i) Early postoperative thrombosis: This can be caused by surgical or by patient-related problems. Low-dose heparin or an antiplatelet agent may be of benefit and a 24- to 48-h heparin infusion immediately after surgery may prevent clotting in high-risk patients.

- Failure of fistula maturation: If the venous segment fails to dilate and develops a thick wall, it cannot be used for dialysis. Possible reasons include:

 (i) Poor surgical technique (with poor anastomosis) or stenosis at the anastomosis with poor flow into the vein.
 (ii) Several tributaries draining the blood and one main venous segment not developing. In this situation, partial ligation of non-fistula tributaries may solve the problem.
(iii) In some patients (including children, older patients, and patients with diabetes mellitus) the fistula may fail to develop for no apparent reason.

- Access in obese patients: In obese patients with a thick subcutaneous layer, the fistula may be difficult to access. Moving the vessels to the subcutaneous area can solve this.

Late failure: This is usually caused by thrombosis or stenosis. A stricture higher up in the venous segment can cause high venous pressure during dialysis and poor flow, with a high rate of recirculation. Stenosis at the anastomosis will reduce inflow to the dialysis blood circuit, causing prepump arterial pressure to be too low. These problems can be diagnosed by fistulography. Surgical removal of the thrombus and correction of any anatomical problem should be attempted immediately upon detection. Any significant delay leads to enlargement and adhesion of the thrombus to the venous wall, requiring a more involved surgery and often more trauma to the vessel wall.

Infection: Wound infection after surgery and infection in the area of needle insertion are common. Needle insertion infection, cellulitis (involving the skin over the fistula), and sepsis are often seen and can usually be treated with appropriate antibiotics. If the fistula is severely infected or if infection recurs, an alternative access may have to be used while the infection is being treated.

Aneurysm: Large aneurysms and/or pseudo-aneurysms are common in long-standing fistulae. Surgical intervention is needed only if the skin over the dilated segments shows signs of pressure changes or if there is a risk of bleeding or thrombosis.

Venous hypertension: This is a complication of side-to-side anastomosis. The high pressure in the venous segment interferes with venous drainage from the hand, causing pain in the thumb or whole hand. If caused by proximal stenosis, this venous ischemia can be corrected by revision of the stenosis, followed by ligation of the distal vein. This preserves the fistula and corrects the problem. If venous hypertension is severe, however, the fistula may have to be removed and other access created.

Steal syndrome: This is associated with paresthesias, pain, skin changes, and muscle wasting. Usually it can be corrected surgically by reducing the blood flow through the fistula.

Cardiac failure: A relatively rare complication, seen in patients with poor myocardial function. In patients with more than one fistula, the large volume of blood being returned to the heart can cause high-output failure. Cardiac output, measured first with the vascular access patent and then repeated with pressure occlusion of the access, can show the influence of the fistula on cardiac output. If the fistula is having a significant effect on cardiac output, it can be moved or the flow can be reduced.

Poor flow: Sometimes the fistula provides poor flow with very high venous or very low arterial pressures in the dialysis circuit. In these circumstances, there is a risk of high recirculation and poor dialysis (see above).

4.1.3 Arteriovenous Graft

If a native venous fistula cannot be created, tubal material can be grafted under the skin between the artery and the vein and used as blood access. Several graft materials (autogenous, heterogenous, and synthetic) have been tried, including saphenous vein, bovine carotid artery, and PTFE. PTFE grafts are the most commonly used, and results with bovine and saphenous vein graft have been less satisfactory.

An AV graft can be created almost anywhere in the arm (or, although this is rare, in the thigh), as a straight tube or as a loop between an artery and an appropriately sized vein. One common location is to insert the graft between the radial artery and the basilic vein; another is to loop the graft between the brachial artery and the basilic vein (see Fig. 4.2). Both the arterial and venous segments where the graft is to be inserted are exposed with separate incisions, and the graft is inserted in a freshly created subcutaneous tunnel with one end sutured to the side of the artery and the other to the side of vein.

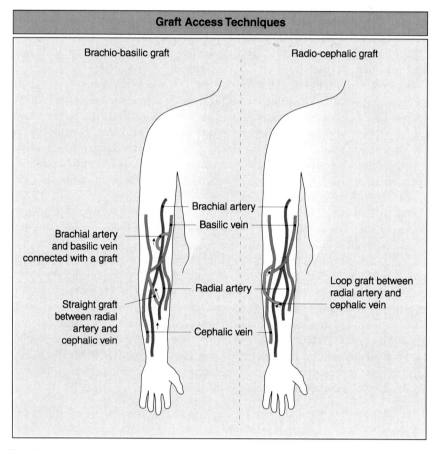

Fig. 4.2 Graft access techniques

4.1.3.1 Graft Use

Grafts have been used immediately after surgical creation but immediate use of grafts may cause extravasations of blood into the tunnel around the graft, leading to compression and graft loss. Infection can also be a risk if a graft is used before wound healing has occurred and edema has subsided. For these reasons, a minimum wait of 1–2 weeks is recommended prior to use.

4.1.3.2 Graft Complications

Some of the complications are similar to those encountered with a fistula. However, AV grafts have more severe problems with infection, stenosis, and thrombosis.

- Infection: This is more common in grafts than in fistulae, particularly in grafts located in the thigh (as many as one quarter of all grafts have problems with infection). A mild infection can be treated with antibiotics, but a severe infection usually requires removal of the graft. Sepsis is a leading cause of morbidity and mortality, and prompt treatment of infection is always warranted.

- Thrombosis and stenosis: Both of these complications are more common in grafts than in fistulae. The most common cause of flow problems is intimal hyperplasia that leads to stenosis at the venous anastomosis. Stenosis of the arterial anastomosis is less common.

4.1.4 Diagnosis and Management of Arteriovenous Dialysis Access

Early detection and correction of access problems are associated with an improved prognosis. Once clinical indicators of a problem are noted, further diagnostic steps must be taken promptly.

4.1.4.1 Clinical Indicators of Problems with Grafts and Fistulae

A reduction in blood flow or a change in thrill or pulsation can indicate an access problem. Similarly, difficulty in placing needles, repeated clotting, excessive bleeding after needle removal, and an unexplained decrease in the dialysis dose (urea reduction ratio) may all suggest problems with the access. Careful palpation and auscultation often suggests a local problem, thus, a sudden increase in the bruit may suggest stenosis. However, these signs are not objective, and more reliable (more sensitive and specific) indicators are:

Dialysis venous pressure: Stenosis or thrombosis at the venous end of a fistula or at the venous anastomosis of a graft is usually associated with increased pressure in the venous segment of the dialysis blood circuit. If venous pressure increases significantly without a change in needle size or blood flow, a flow problem at the venous end of the access must be suspected. Alternatively, if pressure is measured at a blood flow of 200 ml/min, using a 16-gauge needle, a venous pressure consistently >100 mmHg suggests a venous outflow problem. Some investigators have found higher sensitivity and efficacy if a pressure cutoff of 150 mmHg is used [3]. Consistent change in venous pressure over at least three dialyses warrants further investigation. Monitoring of venous pressure without any blood flow (static pressure monitoring) has also been reported to be a good predictor of venous stenosis [4]. This measurement removes the confounding influences of blood flow and other local variables.

Arterial pressure: Difficulty in obtaining the blood flow that the set pump speed demands is associated with very low arterial pressure in the pre-pump segment. This is not as consistent a predictor of a problem as elevated venous pressure, but persistent problems warrant further investigation.

Intra-access pressure and flow relationship: The blood flow in the access is related to pressure and resistance:

$$Q_A = \Delta P/R,$$

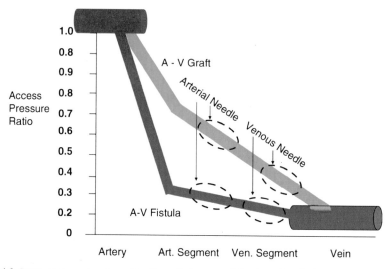

Fig. 4.3 Pressure drop at various sites through the normal fistula and graft (Modified from [5])

where Q_A = access flow; ΔP = pressure difference between the arterial and venous segment; and R = resistance in the access.

The arterial pressure decreases suddenly in the venous segment of the fistula soon after the AV anastomosis even in the absence of any stenosis. The ΔP is about 0.2 (the ratio between arterial and venous pressures). In contrast, the pressure decreases continuously throughout the graft and is generally less than 50% of the systemic pressure (Fig. 4.3).

Increased intra-access pressure thus would decrease the flow rate and this information can be used to detect early problems in the access. Thus, any significant increase in pressure, e.g., >50% of mean arterial pressure (MAP) in a graft may suggest impending problems. Measuring blood flow through the access is a more reliable method for detecting impending problems, any decrease in Q < 750 ml/min, for example, in a graft may suggest a problem. There are many methods of measuring the intra-access pressure and flows but there is no consensus that one is better than the other.

Recirculation: High recirculation (>15%) suggests an access flow problem and dictates further work-up to avoid under-dialysis.

4.1.4.2 Diagnostic Tests

Once an access problem is suspected, several diagnostic alternatives are available. These include Doppler studies, digital subtraction angiography, and traditional angiography.

Doppler studies: Duplex Doppler is a noninvasive technique that can be helpful in diagnosing flow problems such as stenosis. However, a Doppler study does not provide as much anatomical detail of the access as angiography.

Angiography: A radiopaque contrast medium is injected either into the artery close to the anastomosis (vein or graft) or into the distal end of the access. Subsequent radiographic study gives accurate anatomical details of the access and is very useful in determining stenosis, thrombosis, steal syndrome, large run-off, and other problems. When properly carried out, an angiogram is perhaps the most dependable diagnostic procedure, but it is invasive and requires x-ray exposure.

4.1.4.3 Management

Once a problem has been diagnosed as stenosis or thrombosis, either surgical or radiological intervention is needed. The success of the intervention in a clotted access depends on the promptness of intervention. A clotted access must be declotted within 24 h.

Declotting and percutaneous angioplasty: Access declotting and balloon angioplasty by radiological procedures are commonly used, with high initial success rates (up to 90%), but re-stenosis occurs in 50–70% of cases [6]. Stents have been used in cases of restenosis but, in one controlled trial, a metallic endovascular stent afforded no benefit; indeed, the re-stenosis rate may have been higher with it [7]. Better results have been reported with elastic stents, but more experience is needed to assess the efficacy of this technique.

Surgical correction: Surgical correction, particularly of a tight stenosis, remains the gold standard. The need for hospitalization has reduced the use of surgical correction, however, and percutaneous angioplasty is being used more frequently.

Thrombolysis: Early attempts to dissolve clots with the use of streptokinase and urokinase were not very successful. Recently, the use of mechanical and pharmacological agents by pulse spray technique has been reported to lead to 1-year patency rates of 90% [8], but more data are needed to verify the efficacy of this technique. It is important for any venous stenosis to be corrected to prevent reclotting. Thrombolytic agents should be avoided in patients at a high risk of bleeding. Mechanical disruption without the use of any thrombolytic agent has been reported to be as successful [9].

4.1.5 Dual-Lumen Catheters with Dacron Cuff

Tunneled catheters must only be used when no other alternative for dialysis access is available. There must be a plan for the placement of more permanent access and removal of the catheter as soon as possible, because the catheters have higher rates of complications and death. The catheter must not be placed on the same site as the

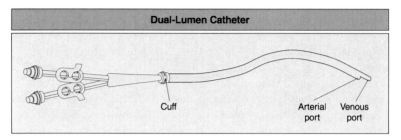

Fig. 4.4 Dual-lumen catheter

maturing fistula or graft. The preferred site for catheter placement is the right internal jugular (IJ). Other sites include the external jugular, the left internal and external jugular, and, if no other alternative is available, only then should the subclavian vein be used. Dual-lumen catheters are implanted surgically into the right atrium through a central (e.g., IJ) vein. It is important to make sure that the tip of the catheter lies in the upper part of the right atrium, even when the patient sits up and the heart drops down. This placement should be verified radiologically. The tip sitting in the superior vena cava leads to lower blood flow and catheter malfunction. Dual-lumen catheters are sometimes used as intermediate-term dialysis access. The extravenous segment of the cuff is tunneled under the skin and the Dacron® (polyester; DuPont Laboratories, Wilmington, DE, USA) cuff is positioned just under the exit site (see Fig. 4.4). A large subcutaneous tissue between the exit and the cuff is a potential site for infection. Several different catheters are available, some of which require a slight modification to the insertion technique, but details of this are beyond the scope of this book [10].

As stated above, these catheters should be used only when access sites that are more permanent are not available. As discussed below, the catheters are associated with higher morbidity, expense, and death. Thus, these catheters should be avoided if possible. Stenosis of the central vein is very common with prolonged use of catheters; subclavian insertion has a higher rate of venous stenosis than IJ insertion.

4.1.5.1 Complications

Complications include immediate surgical complications and late medical complications. Surgical complications are related to the insertion procedure and are discussed in Section 4.2.2. Common late medical complications include infection, clotting of the catheter and vein, poor blood flow, and venous stenosis.

Clotting: Clotting of the catheter and/or its pores is a common and frustrating problem. The most common presentation is inadequate blood flow with abnormal pressure readings in the dialysis circuit. Poor arterial flow is more common than problems with the return of blood through the venous segment. Treatment involves several steps. First, attempts are made to declot the catheter by aspiration of the clots and cleaning of the catheter. If this is not successful (as is often the case), the cleaning attempt is followed by a local infusion of urokinase or streptokinase. Tissue plaminogen activator (tPA) are also being used now. If this fails, a catheterogram can be obtained by infusing radiocontrast material and taking a radiograph. If clots are present, declotting can be attempted under fluoroscopy by an interventional radiologist using a snare technique. If the catheter is still nonfunctional, it may have to be removed and a new one inserted. Clots often occur at the tip of the catheter and may result from poor catheter care. Good technique constitutes that when at the end of the treatment, the catheter is primed with heparin steps are taken to prevent backflow of blood from the vein into the tip. This can be done by clamping the catheter while the syringe is still pushing heparin in and there is enough pressure on the piston to prevent entry of blood into the catheter tip. Thrombosis may follow infection, so prevention of clot formation is important. A kink or acute angle of the catheter in the subcutaneous tunnel will also predispose the catheter to thrombosis and poor flow. Infection: Infections of the exit site, tunnel, cuff, and catheter are common, and catheter-related sepsis can occur in these patients. The rate of infection varies from 2–25%, and *Staphylococcus aureus* and *S. epidermidis* are the organisms most commonly involved.

Exit site infection: Redness and/or purulent discharge around the exit site are signs of infection. Any discharge should be cultured to enable identification of the organism responsible. Exit site infection without cuff involvement can be treated easily with local and/or systemic antibiotics. If pressure on the cuff (by squeezing it between thumb and finger) produces pus through the exit site, the cuff is likely to be involved and will probably require catheter removal.

(i) Tunnel infection: Redness and inflammation of the subcutaneous tunnel is a sign of infection. It is important to determine whether the cuff is involved because, if so, medical treatment is not likely to be successful. Tunnel infection without extensive cuff involvement can be treated with an appropriate antibiotic.

(ii) Catheter infection: Positive blood culture obtained through the catheter. If associated with a systemic manifestation of infection, such as fever or leukocytosis, however, it should be treated as sepsis. Catheter infection has occasionally been treated successfully with antibiotics, but a colonized catheter usually has to be removed.

• Poor blood flow: This is the most common and frustrating problem. A good catheterogram usually shows the cause. This can be a kink in the catheter, an acute angle in the tunnel (causing collapse of the catheter), a clot in the lumen or obstructing the pores, suction (causing the tip to be against the vessel wall), or formation of a fibrin sheath around the outside of the catheter. Mechanical obstruction caused by a kink or collapse can be prevented by proper insertion, thrombosis is discussed in more detail above. If the arterial tip of catheter is directed away from the wall and the catheter is placed at the lower end of the superior vena cava or in the right atrium, suction against the wall can be prevented. A fibrin sheath may form around long-standing catheters, causing flow problems.

Several techniques of stripping this sheath while the catheter remains in situ have been described, but their effectiveness has yet to be proven. Attempts to dissolve these sheaths have usually been unsuccessful, and removal and replacement of the catheter are required in most cases.

- Central venous stenosis: Subclavian vein thrombosis and stenosis have been reported with an incidence of <20–50% following catheterization. The problem tends to manifest as swelling of the arm on the involved side, sometimes associated with discomfort or pain. Stenosis is more common with catheters that are placed on the side of a distal arm fistula or graft. It is unclear, however, whether this increases the risk of development of stenosis, or whether increased venous return through the distal access causes swelling of the arm, revealing stenosis. Because the cause of this complication is unclear, placement of an ipsilateral catheter and a distal fistula or graft should be avoided. Other factors that may precipitate stenosis include repeated trauma to the vessel wall by flapping of the catheter, clot formation between the catheter and the vessel wall, and recurrent infections. It is important to avoid use of a disproportionately large or small catheter relative to the size of the subclavian vein. Because subclavian stenoses seem to be more common than those associated with an IJ catheter (10%), insertion of a catheter through the subclavian vein should be avoided if possible [11].

4.1.6 Special Arteriovenous Shunts

External shunts between a distal artery and vein have been used in the past as dialysis access. Although these are largely of historical value, continued problems with the approach described above, and developing interest in unattended nocturnal dialysis, has led to renewed interest in these shunts. Major advantages of these are that no blood pump is required, making nocturnal unattended dialysis safer, and because there is no need for needle insertion, these may become a more desirable alternative for daily dialysis. However, more information on the risk of infection and thrombosis will have to be obtained before these shunts can be used more commonly.

4.1.6.1 Scribner Shunt

In 1960, Quinton and Scribner developed the AV shunt, making chronic dialysis feasible (see Fig. 4.5). This was the method of access for chronic dialysis for the following 15–20 years. It continued to be used as an important access method until the mid-1970s, after which it was replaced by AV fistulae and grafts. In this technique, the ends of a distal artery and vein are tied around two separate vessel tips made of PTFE (Teflon; DuPont Laboratories). Two silicon tubes are attached to the vessel tips and emerge through a skin exit incision, where they are connected to each other by a PTFE connector. Once the clamps are removed, blood flows from

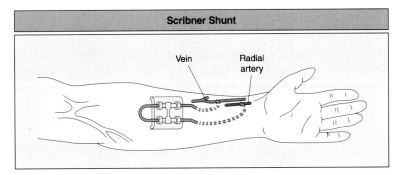

Fig. 4.5 Scribner shunt

the arterial side, through the shunt, and into the vein. For dialysis, the connector is removed and the blood is diverted to the dialysis machine. In between dialysis sessions, the blood flows continuously through the shunt.

4.1.6.2 Thomas Shunt

A silastic tube with a Dacron® skirt is sutured in a major vessel, such as the femoral artery, while another is sutured into the femoral vein. Infection and severe hemorrhage are major complications of this technique.

4.2 Temporary Access

Patients requiring dialysis for a shorter period, such as those with acute reversible renal failure, need temporary access. Additionally, temporary access may be used for patients waiting for permanent access, who require dialysis urgently but for whom peritoneal dialysis (PD) is not suitable, such as for patients with bacteremia or sepsis, in whom permanent access is at risk of infection. Thus, when dialysis is needed urgently or the need is temporary and no other access for dialysis is available, temporary access may be indicated. The advantages of temporary access are that it is easy to insert, typically done at the bedside, the procedure is quick, and vessels needed for a permanent fistula or cannula are preserved. The major disadvantage is the temporary nature, because generally they cannot be used for a prolonged period or used outside of an acute setting. Under appropriate circumstances, with proper technique carried out by an experienced physician, the procedure is relatively safe. However, potentially serious complications can occur. Temporary access uses special dialysis catheters that are inserted into large veins. The most widely used catheters have two lumens—one that gets blood for dialysis (arterial) and another that returns dialyzed blood (venous). Single-lumen catheters, which require a "single needle setup" on the dialysis machine, are also available but are used less frequently. Catheters can be inserted in any one of three commonly used veins: the IJ, subclavian, or femoral.

4.2.1 General Technique

Once the vein to be accessed is identified and the skin site of insertion is selected, some of the technical steps are common to all sites. The procedure can be performed at the bedside under sterile technique, with sterile gowns, gloves, masks, and drapes. The general technique uses the Seldinger method of catheter insertion. Blood vessels can be identified by a portable ultrasound probe. The skin is cleaned and prepared with antiseptic solution (such as iodine) and a local anesthetic is applied to the area. A thin (22-gauge) needle attached to a syringe is advanced toward the vein while gentle suction is applied to the syringe. As soon as venous blood is seen in the syringe, the depth and direction of the needle course is noted, the needle withdrawn, and a larger (18-gauge) needle inserted into the vein (directed toward the flow of blood). Once the vein is accessed, a guide wire is advanced into the vein through the needle (to a distance of 10–15 cm). If the wire does not advance freely, it should be withdrawn and a fresh attempt made. Once the guide wire is in place, the needle is withdrawn and the wire is held in place to prevent its withdrawal. The entry site is then enlarged with a size 11 blade. For a larger, dual-lumen catheter, a dilator is then advanced over the guide wire into the vein—through skin, subcutaneous tissue, and venous wall. The dilator is withdrawn, and if a semi-rigid catheter is used, the catheter is then threaded gently over the guide wire into the vein and positioned at the appropriate level. Use of a softer catheter (which is preferable) requires insertion of a peel-away sheath over the introducer. The introducer (with sheath) is threaded over the guide wire and then withdrawn, leaving the sheath in the vein. The catheter can then be introduced through the sheath, positioned at the appropriate level, the blood flow checked, and the sheath peeled off slowly and withdrawn. Every precaution should be taken to ensure that the catheter does not move out while the sheath is peeled off. The catheter can be fixed to the skin close to the exit point with a suture and filled with heparinized saline to prevent clotting. It is important that the instruction sheet accompanying the catheter is read carefully prior to starting the procedure. After the subclavian or IJ insertion, a chest x-ray must be taken to ensure the location is correct and that no trauma has occurred. Dialysis should not be initiated before this x-ray has been reviewed. The technique differs for different catheters and is discussed extensively in the brochures accompanying the catheters.

4.2.1.1 Internal Jugular Access

Recently, there has been a change from subclavian to IJ access, because this site appears to result in venous stenosis less frequently. A right IJ is preferred (see Fig. 4.6a), because the course on this side is straighter and it is therefore easier to guide the catheter tip into the superior vena cava. On the left side, the presence of the thoracic duct and the fact that the apex of the lung is higher makes entry on this side less desirable.

Insertion involves placing the patient in a supine position with the head lowered at 15–20° and turned away to the left. The IJ can be accessed at three locations:

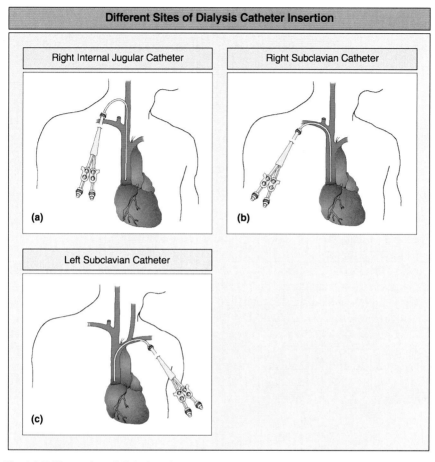

Fig. 4.6 Different sites of dialysis catheter insertion

centrally (the easiest and most common route), anteriorly, or posteriorly. Ultrasonic visualization of the vein prior to placement of these catheters has made the technique much safer, and has become standard practice.

4.2.1.2 Subclavian Access (Least Desirable)

The patient lies supine with their head down and turned away from the operator. The infraclavicular approach is most commonly used, but in difficult patients an experienced operator can use the supraclavicular approach. A thin (22-gauge) needle on a syringe filled with heparinized saline is inserted into the cleaned and anesthetized area under the clavicle (where its medial third joins the lateral two thirds at the lateral aspect of the deltopectoral groove). The needle first touches the inferior margin of the clavicle and is then advanced deeper into the subclavian vein. The use of a thin-gauge needle prevents the formation of a large hole if the needle enters the artery. Gentle suction should be applied to the syringe while advancing the needle. As soon as venous blood can be easily withdrawn, the needle's position and direction are noted and it is withdrawn. A larger bore (18-gauge) needle is then advanced into the vein, the syringe removed, and a guide wire inserted through the needle into the vein. If the 22-gauge needle fails to reach the vein, a longer and larger bore needle can be used. The guide wire should pass easily to the superior vena cava—about 10–15 cm in an average sized adult. If it is difficult to advance the guide wire, it should not be forced but must be withdrawn. The catheter insertion technique is then identical to that discussed in Section 4.2.1 (see Fig. 4.6b and c).

4.2.1.3 Femoral Access

Shaldon first described this relatively safe and easy technique for temporary dialysis access. Compared with subclavian and IJ access, one of the drawbacks of the femoral catheter is the limited mobility the patient experiences because of its insertion location. However, mobility is increased with newer, softer catheters.

The patient lies flat in a supine position with abduction and lateral rotation of the hip and slight flexion of the knee. The area under the inguinal ligament is shaved, cleaned, and prepared. The femoral artery is palpated and the vein (which lies next to it on the medial side) is located, after which, the technique is similar to that described in the general technique section. If the guide wire does not move freely, the wire should be removed completely and the guiding needle reinserted at a flatter angle.

4.2.2 Complications of Temporary Access

Some of the complications related to central catheters are shown in Fig. 4.7 [10]. If a subclavian catheter inserted from the right side perforates the wall of the superior vena cava and enters the pericardial cavity, there is risk of pericardial tamponade when dialysis is started. Immediate cessation of dialysis may save the patient's life (see Fig. 4.7a). A full-sized subclavian catheter inserted from the right side in a small patient may perforate the wall of the right atrium. This injury is nearly always fatal (see Fig. 4.7b). If a right-sided catheter ends up with the tip in contact with the upper part of the wall of the right atrium it may slowly cause the development of a pedunculated ball thrombus. This can obstruct the passage of blood through the tricuspid valve and thus kill the patient (see Fig. 4.7c). A subclavian catheter inserted from the left side may "tent" the right wall of the superior vena cava. The danger is that after one or more dialyses it could perforate the wall (see Fig. 4.7d). In some instances, a catheter that perforates the wall in this way leaves the tip of the catheter in the parenchyma of the lung. There may be no symptoms until the start of dialysis, when the patient will experience profuse bright red hemoptysis (see Fig. 4.7e).

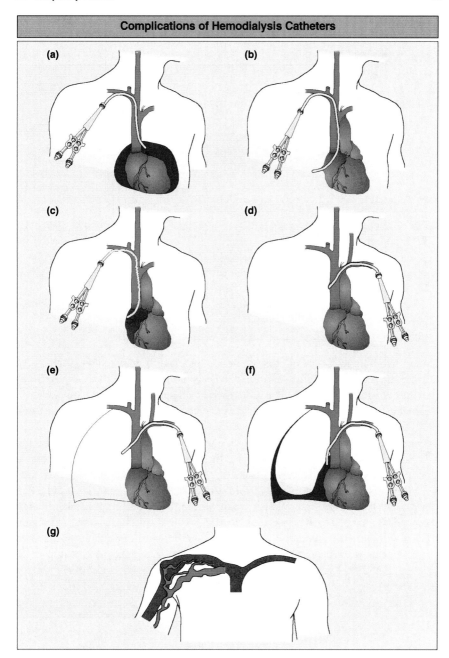

Fig. 4.7 Adapted with permission from [10]

If perforation of the superior vena cava causes blood to track down into the right hemithorax, continuation of dialysis may result in death (see Fig. 4.7f). If subclavian vein thrombosis is not detected early, it will become permanent and essentially untreatable. Tell-tale collateral veins will be seen coursing over the shoulder (see Fig. 4.7g). Acute catheter complications can be divided into two major categories: immediate procedure-related complications, and late complications.

4.2.2.1 Procedure-Related Complications of Superior Vena Cava Access (Subclavian and Internal Jugular)

These procedure-related complications include:

Puncture of the accompanying artery
Pneumothorax
Hemothorax
Pneumo-hemothorax (with subclavian access)
Injury to the brachial plexus (with subclavian access)
Pericardial hemorrhage or mediastinal hemorrhage (with vena caval injury and puncture)
Puncture of right atrium

Cardiac arrhythmias. Some of these complications are life threatening, so the situation must be reviewed carefully before dialysis is initiated. Only after an initial chest x-ray has been reviewed and the results found to be normal should a subclavian or IJ catheter be used for dialysis. Arterial puncture usually means that the location and/or the direction of the needle is incorrect—sometimes the anatomy is different to that expected. To avoid this, the insertion technique should be followed carefully and a fine probe needle used to minimize the bleeding that results from accidental puncture of an artery. If the artery is punctured, the needle should be withdrawn and firm local pressure applied for 15–20 min. If the catheter or dilator has accidentally been placed in an artery, it should be withdrawn, local pressure applied, and dialysis postponed or changed to the opposite side. If urgent dialysis is necessary, this should be done without anticoagulation. A large pneumothorax or hemothorax usually requires insertion of a chest tube. Injury to the superior vena cava or atrium is life threatening and may require surgical intervention. If the patient develops arrhythmias, chest pain, or persistent hypotension, dialysis must be stopped immediately, an investigation started, and a surgeon alerted.

4.2.2.2 Procedure-Related Complications of Femoral Vein Catheters

The most common complication is puncture of the femoral artery. This should be managed in the manner described above. It is not advisable to dialyze using a dual-lumen dialysis catheter in the femoral artery. Severe trauma to the femoral vein can also occur with a large hemorrhage; major damage to the femoral nerve is unusual.

4.2.2.3 Late Complications

Late complications include infection, thrombosis, and stenosis. Infection is more common with the femoral catheter than with subclavian or IJ catheters. These complications are similar to those discussed earlier in the permanent catheter section.

4.2.3 Comparison of the Three Access Sites

Of the three access sites, insertion of a catheter in the subclavian vein requires the most experience, is most difficult, and is associated with the most serious complications. It is technically difficult and should not be attempted in the presence of acute respiratory distress or pulmonary edema. However, once inserted, this site is the most stable and allows the patient substantial mobility. Patients with bacteremia should not be given a subclavian catheter, because the risk of colonization is high. Formation of subclavian venous stricture is common and, for this reason, its prolonged use must be discouraged.

It is technically easier to insert a catheter into the right IJ site, and there are fewer complications. This can be attempted in patients with respiratory distress, can be used for weeks, and has a lower incidence of venous stricture and stenosis. However, unless the catheter is anchored properly and secured firmly, the catheter interferes with mobility. The infection rate is similar to that observed with subclavian catheters.

The femoral site is easily used, even by an operator with limited skills, and can be used in almost any patient, even those who have bacteremia. Use of the femoral site is associated with a lower frequency of complications, and life-threatening complications are seldom encountered. The major drawbacks of this technique are limited patient mobility and an increased risk of infection. Because of these issues, this site should not be used for prolonged periods, and the catheter should be changed frequently.

Vascular access for hemodialysis remains one of the most formidable challenges in the management of the end-stage renal disease (ESRD) patient. The costs associated with access problems are very high in financial, emotional, and medical terms. Among current techniques, the AV fistula is the gold standard, and every attempt should be made to create an AV fistula in every patient. Catheters have several major complications and should be avoided when possible. The success of future advances in dialysis technique, whether in the form of daily dialysis or a wearable artificial kidney, will depend largely on better blood access techniques than those currently available.

4.3 Impact of Access

Vascular access accounts for one third of all hospitalization in hemodialysis patients and, in the first year, as much as 50% of all hospitalizations. Fistula is the

Hospitalization Rate

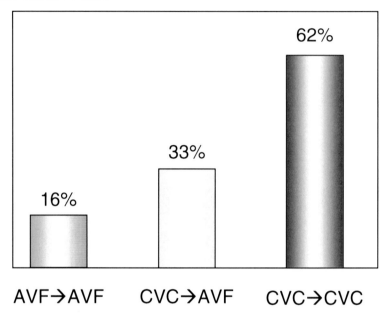

Fig. 4.8 Hospitalization rates associated with different types of vascular access. CVC = central venous catheter, AVF = arterio-venous fistula (Ortega et al: Neph Dial Transpl 20:598, 2005)

gold standard, the hospitalization rate and the relative risk of death being significantly lower in patients with fistula than catheters (Figs. 4.8 and 4.9). Similarly, the cost is lower with a fistula than with a catheter, and presence of an access surveillance program reduces access complications such as thrombosis compared with the absence of such a program (Fig. 4.10).

4.3.1 Access Surveillance

Surveillance could be clinical, instrumental, or a combination of the two. Inability to get enough blood for dialysis within the safe lines pressure limits or a clotted access often forces further work up, however, the goal of a good program is to intervene prior to occurrence of these terminal events. A reduced dose of dialysis, increased recirculation, change in flow and pressure relationship, changes in characteristics of bruit over the access, development of swelling, and infection are some of the clinical tools used to monitor the access. However, every program should have well-defined monitoring. Static venous pressure, pressure in the venous drip chamber while the blood pump is stopped, is often used for assessing and monitoring the vascular

Access & Mortality

- Mortality Related to Access
- Mortality Related to Type of Access
  - Highest with CVC; - Lowest with AVF:
    - RRD 2.3 CVC vs. AVF

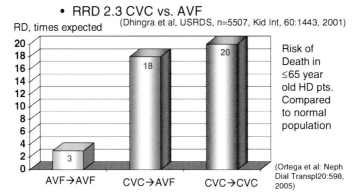

Fig. 4.9 Risk of death with types of access

Prospective Surveillance & prompt Rx of Graft Stenosis Reduces Thrombosis

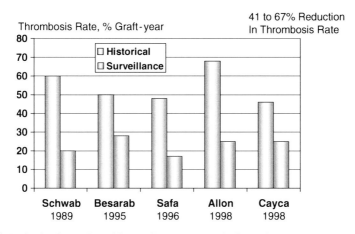

Fig. 4.10 Reduction in clotting with surveillance program in five series

access. Dynamic venous pressure, pressure in the venous drip chamber at a low blood flow of 200 ml/min, is monitored for each run. This pressure, corrected for the needle size and hematocrit, seems to be a good easy monitoring tool for impending problems. Venous pressure of >120 mmHg for 15-gauge needles and >150 mmHg for 16-gauge needles for three dialysis sessions suggests further investigation.

Several methods to monitor access flows are available in the market but their value has not been proven. Static pressure monitoring seems to be a more sensitive method with less confounding variables.

References

1. Anonymous. Clinical practice guidelines for vascular access. National Kidney Foundation-Dialysis Outcomes Quality Initiative. *Am J Kid Dis* 1997, 30(Suppl 3):S154–S191.
2. Rubens F, Wellington JL. Brachiocephalic fistula: A useful alternative for vascular access in chronic hemodialysis. *Cardiovasc Surg* 1993, 1:128–130.
3. Schwab SJ, Raymond JR, Saeed M et al. Prevention of fistula thrombosis: Early detection of venous stenosis. *Kidney Int* 1989, 36:707–711.
4. Besarab A, Sullivan K, Ross R et al. Utility of intra-access pressure monitoring in detecting and correcting venous outlet stenosis prior to thrombosis. *Kidney Int* 1995, 47:1364–1673.
5. Besarab A, Frinak S, Aslam M: Pressure measurements in the surveillance of vascular accesses. In Gray R (ed): A Multidisciplinary Approach for Hemodialysis Access. Philadelphia, PA, Lippincott Williams & Wilkins, 2002, Chapter 21, pp. 137–150.
6. Windus DW. Permanent vascular access: a nephrologist's view. *Am J Kidney Dis* 1993, 21:457–471.
7. Beathard G. Gianturco self-expanding stents in the treatment of stenosis in dialysis access grafts. *Kidney Int* 1993, 43:872–877.
8. Valji K, Bookstein JJ, Roberts AC et al. Pharmacomechanical thrombolysis and angioplasty in the management of clotted graft. Early and late clinical results. *Radiology* 1991, 178:243–247.
9. Trerotola SO, Lund GB, Scheel PJ et al. Thrombosed dialysis access grafts: percutaneous mechanical declotting without urokinase. *Radiology* 1994, 191:721–726.
10. Uldall R. Hemodialysis access. Part A: Temporary. In *Replacement of Renal Function by Dialysis, 4th Edition.* Edited by C Jacobs, CM Kjellstrand, KM Koch and JF Winchester. Dordrecht: Kluwer Academic Publishers, 1996:277–293.
11. Hernández D, Díaz F, Rufino M et al. Subclavian vascular access stenosis in dialysis patients: natural history and risk factors. *J Am Soc Nephrol* 1998, 9:1507–1510.

Chapter 5
Complications of Hemodialysis

Complications of hemodialysis can be divided into two major groups:

– Treatment-related medical complications: There are frequent intradialytic complications, these (in order of frequency) include hypotension, muscle cramps, nausea and vomiting, flushing of face, headache, increased pruritus, chest pain, fever, and chills.
– Machine-related complications: These complications are due to accidents or failure of safety mechanisms of hemodialysis treatment. They include air embolism, hemolysis, hyperthermia or hypothermia, blood loss, and conductivity problems.

5.1 Medical Complications

5.1.1 Hypotension

Hypotension occurs in 15–40% of dialyses and is the most common intradialytic complication. It is more common in patients being dialyzed with acetate dialysate than in those using bicarbonate-containing dialysate.

The pathogenesis is multifactorial, complex, and poorly understood. However, many of the contributing factors are known, and understanding of these can help to reduce the frequency and severity of hypotension (see Table 5.1). During hemodialysis, blood is exposed to a foreign surface, excess body fluid is removed by ultrafiltration (UF), substances move from the dialysate into the blood, and there is a decrease in plasma solutes (in particular those with a low molecular weight) as a result of diffusion. Hypotension appears to be related to the body's response to these three processes.

S. Ahmad, *Manual of Clinical Dialysis*, DOI 10.1007/978-0-387-09651-3_5,
© Springer Science+Business Media LLC 2009

Table 5.1 Common corrective treatment steps for intradialytic hypotension

Action	Comments
Reduce blood flow	Questionable benefit
Lower UFR	UFR can be stopped if BP remains low
Trendelenberg position	Increases cerebral perfusion and reduces risk of aspiration
Restore plasma volume	Use normal saline 100–250 ml
Give nasal oxygen 2–4 l/min	Prevention of hypoxemia is helpful
Pressor agents	Useful in acute but not in chronic setting
Discontinue dialysis	Rarely needed

5.1.1.1 Effect of Ultrafiltration

Salt intake with consequent drinking of water leads to the accumulation of fluid between two dialysis treatments, this causes primarily the expansion of extracellular fluid (ECF), with some expansion of intracellular fluid (ICF) associated with free water excess. This extra fluid contributes to hypertension and other clinical sequelae. The fluid excess is removed by UF and some sodium excess by diffusion during dialysis. Direct access to the vascular space means that the fluid and Na is removed from the plasma space, a smaller subcompartment of the ECF. With the drop in plasma volume (PV) and plasma Na, both water and Na move from the extravascular compartments of ECF into the plasma. Hypotension will result if the fluid removal from the plasma compartment is at a faster rate than the reequilibration rate into the plasma, leading to PV depletion (see Fig. 5.1). The movement into the PV is governed by the Starling's forces and, under normal conditions, the reequilibration rate into the plasma is 15–25 ml/kg/h. Thus, a UF rate (UFR) faster than the reequilibration rate would cause hypotension.

- Reduction in PV: A significant reduction in PV leads to cardiac under filling and subsequent hypotension. Several factors during dialysis can lead to the depletion of PV:

  (i) Rapid UF: Use of dialyzers with a high K_{uf} and shorter duration of dialysis often leads to a rapid UF rate. A patient who gains, for example, 4 kg in fluid weight between dialyses would have about 1 l of this excess fluid in the PV and the remainder in the extravascular space (the largest component of it being in the interstitial space). As the PV decreases with UF, extravascular fluid moves into the vascular space (secondary to the Starling forces) and the entire 4 l of excess fluid can be removed via the plasma space. However, if the UFR is greater than the rate at which the fluid moves into the vascular space, the PV is decreased, even though there is excess fluid in the extravascular space—leading to hemodynamic instability and hypotension (see Fig. 5.1). In a stable dialysis patient without other risk factors, a UFR of <20 ml/kg/h is generally well tolerated. A UFR greater than this, particularly in patients at risk for hemodynamic instability, invariably leads to hypotension. This scenario can

Fig. 5.1 Despite the patient in the lower example having more fluid volume than the patient in the upper example, hypotension is more likely; the ultrafiltration rate (UFR) is higher than the rate at which the extracellular fluid can enter the plasma volume (PV) and so the PV will decline, leading to hypotension. *ICV* intracellular volume, *ECV* extracellular volume

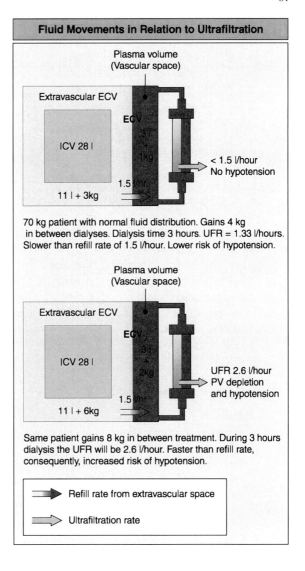

Fluid Movements in Relation to Ultrafiltration

70 kg patient with normal fluid distribution. Gains 4 kg in between dialyses. Dialysis time 3 hours. UFR = 1.33 l/hours. Slower than refill rate of 1.5 l/hour. Lower risk of hypotension.

Same patient gains 8 kg in between treatment. During 3 hours dialysis the UFR will be 2.6 l/hour. Faster than refill rate, consequently, increased risk of hypotension.

Refill rate from extravascular space

Ultrafiltration rate

be avoided by educating the patient about weight gain and about the rate of UF and its consequences. In high-risk patients, slower and longer dialysis will reduce the risk of hypotension.

Interdialytic Weight Gain (IDWG): Large interdialytic weight gain (IDWG) is the main cause of rapid UF. It has been clearly shown that the sodium intake, not water intake, is the major cause of large IDWG [13]. Thus, patient counseling should emphasize limiting the daily sodium intake, usually to about 2 g per day.

(ii) Slower refilling of plasma space: Two major groups of factors influence the rate of refilling of the plasma space from the extravascular space. The first of these are Starling forces, which (along with capillary permeability) govern the movement of fluid between the vascular and interstitial spaces. Starling forces, which reduce the rate of refilling of the vascular space, include hypoalbuminemia, right-sided heart failure, increased permeability of the capillary membrane (capillary leak syndrome), and increased hydrostatic pressure in the capillaries. The commonly used antihypertensive dihydropyridine calcium channel blockers dilate the precapillary sphincter thus increasing the intracapillary pressure and reducing the reequilibration rate. Similarly, other antihypertensive medications, by modifying the normal responses to UF, may limit the ability to adequate UF and volume control. Osmolar factors are the other cause of slower filling. During dialysis, the plasma and ECF osmolarity decline due to the diffusion of solutes. Rapid dialysis using hypotonic dialysate (relative to plasma) leads to a rapid decline in plasma osmolarity, to a reduced rate of PV refilling, and to hypotension. This happens when the sodium concentration of the dialysate is appreciably lower than that of the plasma (in excess of 4 mEq/l). This causes a drop in plasma osmolarity and water may move into the extravascular (interstitial and intracellular) spaces until a new equilibrium is reached. At this time, a patient undergoing UF may have a rapid reduction in PV and be at risk of hypotension. After a new steady state is reached, UF starts refilling the PV; however, during the dialysis period, the patient is at risk. This risk can be reduced by avoiding UF during the first hour or so of dialysis if the plasma sodium concentration is >4 mEq/l higher than the dialysate sodium concentration. Alternatively, dialysate with a higher osmolarity can be used if feasible.

- Reduction in ECF: Significant ECF depletion leads to hemodynamic instability and hypotension [1]. This is commonly encountered under two scenarios.
- Dry weight estimation problems: If a patient's dry weight (body weight minus water weight) has been underestimated (its overestimation is a more common problem), attempts to reduce the weight to this level will result in significant intradialytic morbidity. Ignoring the changes in tissue weight is more common. Typically, when a patient who has been uremic and anorexic initiates dialysis, appetite and well-being improve gradually and tissue mass increases. If dry weight is not increased, this patient will have problems with hemodynamic instability.

(iii) Osmolar effects: As discussed previously, the osmolarity of ECF gradually declines during dialysis. This osmolar decline can affect hemodynamic stability by altering ECF volume and vascular resistance.

It has been proposed that movement of water from the ECF into the intracellular space reduces the ECF beyond the level of reduction caused by UF. Thus, the excessive reduction in ECF during dialysis, because of a combination of UF and flux into the cells, causes hypotension. Once dialysis is stopped, however, the ECF is repleted slowly and the patient continues to have ECF excess.

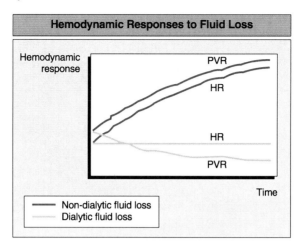

Fig. 5.2 *PVR* peripheral vascular resistance, *HR* heart rate

The normal response to PV and ECF reductions is an increase in heart rate and vascular resistance. These responses prevent a decline in blood pressure (BP) (see Fig. 5.2). The response to UF during dialysis is, however, abnormal; heart rate increase is inadequate, the increase in vascular resistance is blunted [2], and there may even be a decrease in vascular resistance. Possible factors influencing these responses are discussed below. It has been suggested that a decrease in osmolarity is responsible for the abnormality of the vascular resistance. This inappropriate response may also be a result of an abnormality of the autonomic system.

As discussed above, the normal vascular response to UF (an increase in vascular resistance) is not seen during dialysis. The decrease in PV during dialysis leads to decreased cardiac filling and output. Any decrease in vascular resistance allows pooling of blood in the venous system, lowering BP (which is a product of cardiac output and vascular resistance) and increasing the risk of hypotension. There are multiple causes of the abnormal response of the vascular resistance. The possible relationship between osmolarity and vascular resistance and the effect of increased temperature have been discussed above, while other factors are listed below:

– Autonomic dysfunction: This is common in patients with diabetes and in older patients. It contributes to the inability to increase vascular resistance and heart rate and increases the risk of hypotension. Few reports suggest that the use of serotonin uptake inhibitor, sertraline (4- to 6-week trial), improves intradialytic hypotension (Fig. 5.3); sertraline is suggested to improve autonomic function.
– An alpha adrenergic agonist, ten mg dose of midodrine, given 2 h before dialysis has also been reported to reduce hypotensive episodes.
– Anemia: Prior to the use of erythropoeitin (Epo), most patients suffered from severe anemia, which, in turn, caused vasodilation and placed the patients at increased risk of hypotension. Anemia does not, however, appear to be a factor when Epo is used.

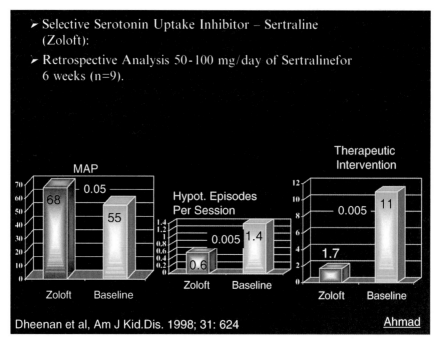

Fig. 5.3 The improvement in intra-dialytic blood pressure and reduced interventions with sertraline (Zoloft) compared to without it (Baseline)

- Production of vasodepressors: During dialysis, there are indications that certain vasodepressors (such as adenosine) are produced from hypoperfused tissues. Because norepinephrine release is impaired in uremia, the vasodilation caused by adenosine is unchecked and a vicious cycle of hypotension and tissue ischemia is initiated. Calcitonin-related gene factor is another vasodepressor that may be produced during dialysis, although more work in this area is needed to confirm this. These vasodepressors are relatively large molecules and are not readily removed by diffusion dialysis.
- Acetate dialysate: Acetate is a vasodilator and, as such, its accumulation in the blood causes hypotension. Although current bicarbonate dialysate does not have large concentration of acetate, most dialysate still contain 4–8 mEq/l acetate, and evidence suggests that even relatively smaller concentration such as 10 mEq/l may cause significant hypotension (2a). Evidence is also accumulating that even as small as 3 mEq/l of acetate may cause cytokine production that, in turn, potentially contributes to intradialytic hemodynamic instability.

  • Production of cytokines: The cellulosic membrane of dialyzers causes complement activation and generation of cytokines (including interleukins). It has been speculated that these cytokines are responsible for an abnormal vascular response but the issue remains controversial.

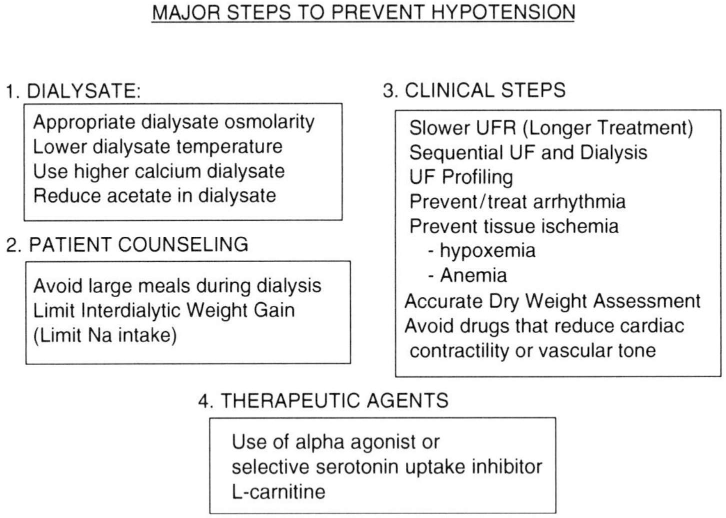

MAJOR STEPS TO PREVENT HYPOTENSION

1. DIALYSATE:

Appropriate dialysate osmolarity
Lower dialysate temperature
Use higher calcium dialysate
Reduce acetate in dialysate

2. PATIENT COUNSELING

Avoid large meals during dialysis
Limit Interdialytic Weight Gain
(Limit Na intake)

3. CLINICAL STEPS

Slower UFR (Longer Treatment)
Sequential UF and Dialysis
UF Profiling
Prevent/treat arrhythmia
Prevent tissue ischemia
 - hypoxemia
 - Anemia
Accurate Dry Weight Assessment
Avoid drugs that reduce cardiac
 contractility or vascular tone

4. THERAPEUTIC AGENTS

Use of alpha agonist or
selective serotonin uptake inhibitor
L-carnitine

Fig. 5.4 Major steps to prevent hypotension

- Cardiac disease: Myocardial dysfunction is common in dialysis patients and might be an important contributor to abnormal cardiac and vascular response. This is discussed in detail below.
- Use of antihypertensive medications: Antihypertensive drugs can blunt the normal response to volume contraction. If they must be used, it is better to use short-acting agents that can be withheld on the day of dialysis. Withholding long-acting medications is ineffective.

Myocardial diseases and dysfunction are prevalent among dialysis patients and left ventricular hypertrophy (LVH), diastolic dysfunction, myocardial contractility problems, and systolic dysfunction are common, as is coronary artery disease. Because of cardiac disease, coupled with fluid and electrolyte shifts, cardiac arrhythmias during dialysis are not unusual. Because hypotension may decrease myocardial perfusion and oxygenation (which may lead to cardiac arrhythmias, leading to more severe hypotension), it is particularly important to take all necessary steps to minimize hypotension in patients with cardiac complications. Preventing and aggressively treating hypotension and/or arrhythmias should break this vicious cycle (see Fig. 5.4).

5.1.1.2 Prevention of Hemodynamic Instability

- Sequential UF and dialysis: UF reduces ECF, and diffusion dialysis reduces osmolarity. The separation of the UF and diffusion processes prevents the osmolar shift that occurs while UF is reducing ECF, whereas the cessation of UF while dialysis is reducing the osmolarity of ECF prevents a decrease in ECF volume. The main drawback of sequential ultrafiltration (SUF) is the prolongation of treatment.

- Higher osmolarity dialysate (sodium modeling): Use of dialysate with a higher sodium concentration, while preventing a decline in osmolarity, later followed by a lowering of dialysate sodium to bring down the serum sodium has been used and termed as sodium modeling or ramping. Sodium modeling has been proposed in order to achieve more stable dialysis. At the start of dialysis, dialysate sodium is raised to 145 mEq/l and after a period it is decreased to 135 mEq/l [3]. Various rates of sodium decline (linear to multiple steps) have been used to reduce intradialytic hemodynamic instability and hypotension. The main drawback of this method is the potential for positive sodium balance and its consequences. Improper use of dialysate sodium concentrations would lead to an undesirable increase in the sodium content of the ECF. Increased thirst and water intake leads to the movement of water from the intracellular fluid (ICF) causes expansion of ECF soon after dialysis ceases. Long-term effects of this technique have not been widely evaluated. There is some indication of sodium accumulation, ECV excess, and hypertension. It is important to ensure that these do not occur because they have an adverse effect on survival.
- Dialysate temperature: Higher dialysate temperature increases body temperature, which, in turn causes vasodilation and may lead to hypotension. Conversely, lower dialysate temperature (36.0–36.5°C) has been shown to increase hemodynamic stability and decrease episodes of hypotension [4]. It is important to note that some patients feel cold and/or are uncomfortable at these lower temperatures. Although it has been suggested that this decrease in temperature does not affect tissue perfusion and movement of solutes (including uremic toxins), more work is needed to ensure that it does not have an adverse effect on dialysis efficiency.

5.1.1.3 Clinical Manifestation of Hypotension

Intradialytic hypotension may present as signs/symptoms of vascular insufficiency including feeling unwell, dizziness, cramps, nausea, sweating, and, in severe cases, complete collapse and unresponsiveness. Others may not exhibit symptoms until BP declines to a dangerous level. To avoid serious complications, BP should be monitored frequently. This task has been simplified by the widespread use of automatic BP-monitoring devices and frequent readings (e.g., every 15 min) can be taken in patients at high risk.

5.1.1.4 Treatment of Hypotension

Some of the management steps directed toward prevention of hypotensive episodes have been discussed previously. Once hypotension is detected, the treatment depends on its severity. Common corrective measures include:

- Reducing blood flow: This traditional practice is of questionable benefit. With older non-volumetric-controlled machines, a slower blood flow through the dialyzer reduced the UF rate by decreasing pressure on the blood side, which, in turn, lowered the transmembrane pressure (TMP). However, modern volumetric controls maintain a desired TMP for the desired UFR, independent of Qb. A slower blood flow does reduce the diffusion of solutes, which may help to reduce the rate of accumulation of acetate (if acetate dialysate is used). In addition, the slowing of diffusion reduces the rate of osmolar decline and may therefore prevent the hypotension that is caused by a rapid drop in serum osmolarity (or sodium concentration). It is important to remember that the slowing of dialysis will affect the dialysis dose by reducing the removal of toxin(s), and the impact of this should be given serious consideration. Thus, automatic reduction of Qb may not be very effective and may have undesirable consequences.
- Reducing UFR: A reduction in BP warrants a reduction in UFR. If the decline in BP is significant, the UFR should be reduced to zero and the situation monitored carefully. Often this alone will stabilize BP and allow the UFR to be increased slowly.
- Trendelenburg position: The patient should be placed in a head-down position to maintain cerebral perfusion and prevent aspiration should the patient start vomiting. If the decline in BP is significant and not responsive to the above measures, additional corrective measures are required.
- Restoration of PV: The most effective treatment of hypotension is expansion of PV, using volume expanders such as normal saline (100- to 250-ml bolus) or albumin solution (in patients with significant hypoalbuminemia). The former is the first choice, because, in patients who have normal albumin levels or very slight hypoalbuminemia, the use of albumin is expensive and not more effective. Hypertonic saline does not appear to be any more effective than normal saline.
- Treatment of hypoxemia: Hypoxemia can contribute to the hemodynamic instability and can cause cardiac arrhythmias. Oxygen, administered nasally, is helpful in such cases.
- Pressor agents: Severely ill, hospitalized patients may already be receiving pressor agents (such as dopamine or norepinephrine), and increasing their rate of infusion can treat hypotension. In a normal dialysis setting, these agents do not have a major role.
- Discontinuation of dialysis: If severe hypotension is persistent and refractory, and severe complications (such as seizures or myocardial damage) are imminent, the patient should be taken off dialysis. This situation is very rare and usually associated with other underlying conditions.

5.1.1.5 Convective vs Diffusive Transport and Hypotension

Compared with traditional diffusion dialysis, convective dialysis techniques such as hemofiltration are associated with less hemodynamic instability and fewer hypotensive episodes. Possible explanations for this include:

– Less-rapid decline in serum osmolarity with convective transport.
– Better clearance of larger molecular weight substances: It has been proposed that certain larger molecules are vasodepressants; therefore, because their clearance is better with hemofiltration, hypotension is less common.
– Lower temperature: Replacement fluids are often not warmed during hemofiltration. Therefore, blood temperature may be lower, preventing vasodilation.
– Use of biocompatible membrane: Hemofiltration typically uses synthetic membranes, which are more permeable, more biocompatible, and are associated with less complement activation and cytokine production.
– No dialysate: In traditional dialysis, the dialysate may not be sterile, and pyrogen-free contaminants can pass across the membranes, thus contributing to hypotension. Because hemofiltration does not use any dialysate, this is not a problem.

5.1.2 Cardiac Arrhythmias

The leading cause of sudden death during dialysis (accounting for 80% of all sudden deaths [5]) is cardiac arrhythmia (both atrial and ventricular). The main causes of this are the presence of coronary artery disease and LVH. It is important to understand that hypotension and arrhythmias are part of a vicious cycle (see Fig. 5.5). In high-risk patients with poor myocardial function and coronary disease,

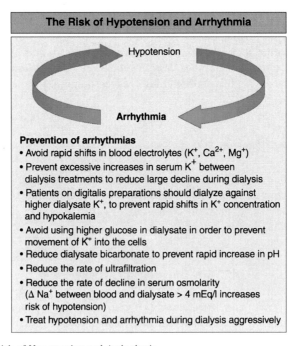

Fig. 5.5 The Risk of Hypotension and Arrhythmia

the prevention, early detection, and management of both arrhythmias and hypotension are very important. The dialytic process may play a contributory role if major fluctuations in electrolytes, pH, and fluid volume are allowed. Thus, dialyzing against a potassium-free fluid using a high-flux dialyzer is inadvisable in a patient with cardiac dysfunction and/or on digitalis. In patients at risk of arrhythmias, calcium and/or potassium modeling may be helpful. Arrhythmias are more prevalent with acetate dialysate than with bicarbonate dialysate.

5.1.3 Intradialytic Hypertension

An increase in BP during the later part of or after dialysis, although less common than hypotension, is sometimes encountered (occurrence estimated to be about 8%) [6]. The exact pathophysiology remains unknown but various mechanisms have been proposed.

Overestimation of dry weight (true dry weight lower than prescribed) appears to be the most common cause of this complication. If a trend toward an increase in BP is observed before the true dry weight is reached, it is mistakenly assumed that the patient is "too dry." It is not uncommon for staff to stop UF or to administer PV expanders to maintain an erroneously high dry weight. This practice should be discouraged because this practice can lead to ECV excess, persistent interdialytic hypertension, use of polypharmacy to control elevated BP, and poor long-term survival. Experience indicates that careful use of UF to reach the correct dry weight will eventually break the cycle of interdialytic and intradialytic hypertension.

Other factors that may contribute to intradialytic hypertension are:

– Decrease in potassium: Intradialytic fall in potassium may stimulate renin or may have direct hemodynamic effect
– Use of beta-adrenergic blockers
– Calcium fluctuation: Increase in calcium may also contribute to hypertension
– Sympathetic stimulation
– Presence of native kidneys
– Use of Epo
– Removal of antihypertensive medications during dialysis

5.1.4 Muscle Cramps

Painful, prolonged, involuntary skeletal muscle contractions (cramps) are a common intradialytic complication. Typically, these occur toward the end of dialysis, may be associated with hypotension (although not always), and respond to treatment with PV expanders. For these reasons, it is thought that cramps are caused by PV depletion. Cramps that are independent of obvious volume depletion and hypotension and that respond in a positive manner to hypertonic saline, mannitol, and hyperosmolar dextrose solution may, however, suggest a role for hypoosmolarity in the pathogenesis of cramps. Presence of peripheral vascular disease is also often associated with muscle cramps.

5.1.4.1 Prevention

– Avoid excessive interdialytic weight gain because rapid removal of large volumes is often complicated by cramps. The patient should be educated about limiting weight gain by limiting sodium intake.
– Prevent hypotension, because steps taken to achieve this are often effective in preventing cramps.
– Avoid excessive UF, which can lead to prolonged, painful cramps.
– Avoid hypomagnesemia (associated with muscle cramps and possibly contributed to by a decline of serum magnesium). In patients with a lower magnesium concentration, a higher concentration of magnesium in the dialysate should be used.

Use medications such as quinine sulfate (which decreases the excitability of motor endplates and can be used to prevent muscle cramps). This is most effective if administered as a single oral dose of 325 mg about 2 h prior to dialysis. Administration of 5–10 mg oxazepam about 2 h prior to dialysis also is effective in relaxing muscles and preventing cramps. Administration of 140 IU vitamin E has also been found to be helpful in reducing cramps.

• Use sodium modeling, because sodium variation during dialysis has been reported to be effective in reducing muscle cramps. However, extreme care must be used to avoid persistent volume expansion.
• A diagnostic work-up to exclude peripheral vascular disease should also be performed.

5.1.4.2 Treatment

Hypertonic saline or dextrose solutions are usually effective in the management of cramps. Oxygen, administered nasally, has also been shown to be useful. Local heat application and muscle stretching is also helpful.

5.1.5 Carnitine and Intradialytic Hypotension, Arrhythmias, and Muscle Cramps

Abnormal carnitine metabolism and profile are prevalent among dialysis patients (see Fig. 5.6) [7]. Carnitine plays an essential role in the cellular energetics of skeletal muscle (particularly cardiac muscles) and the use of L-carnitine supplementation

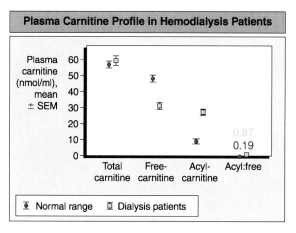

Fig. 5.6 *Acyl-carnitine* acylated carnitine, *Acyl:free* ratio of acylated carnitine:free carnitine, *SEM* standard error of the mean (adapted from [7] with permission)

in this population has been associated with significant reductions in muscle cramps, hypotensive episodes, and intradialytic arrhythmias [8,9]. Not all studies have been controlled and double blinded (some have been anecdotal experiences), but there is enough data to support serious consideration of the use of carnitine in the management of these complications, particularly in patients resistant to conventional therapies. The commonly used 1 g carnitine dose (intravenously) after each dialysis has been effective in hemodialysis patients (although sometimes a larger dosage is administered), whereas in peritoneal dialysis (PD) patients, 1 g carnitine/day (oral) in three divided doses has been used.

5.1.6 Nausea and Vomiting

Nausea and vomiting are common and are often associated with hypotension. Usually, treatment of the hypotension relieves the nausea, and nonresponsive patients can be given anti-emetics. Some patients have excessive secretion of gastric acid during dialysis treatment, which causes severe nausea and sometimes even vomiting. Use of H_2 receptor antagonists or a proton pump inhibitor prior to the start of dialysis is usually very effective for treatment of these symptoms.

5.1.7 Headache

Headache is a common complication and usually has a multifactorial pathogenesis. If associated with hypotension, its management will be similar to the management of hypotension discussed above. Headache in some patients may be caused by a reduction in caffeine levels (caffeine withdrawal) during dialysis. Headache could also be a symptom of dialysis disequilibrium, which is discussed below. In difficult headache cases, a slower shift in osmolarity, electrolytes, and pH, and the use of bicarbonate should all be tried.

5.1.8 Serious, Less Common Complications

5.1.8.1 Dialysis Disequilibrium Syndrome

Dialysis disequilibrium syndrome (DDS) is a disorder of the central nervous system. With recent improvements in dialysis and early institution of dialysis, DDS has become less common but can present as nausea, vomiting, headache, restlessness, vision disturbances, disorientation, and tremors. More serious manifestations include seizures, obtundation, and coma. DDS usually occurs toward the end of or after the termination of dialysis. It tends to be self-limiting, with a complete recovery, which occurs slowly.

The pathogenesis of DDS is unclear, but it is thought to be caused by a rapid shift of plasma osmolarity and/or of plasma pH. A rapid decline in plasma osmolarity in severe uremia could shift water into brain cells—causing swelling and DDS. Similarly, a rapid rise in blood bicarbonate in a severely acidotic patient may cause a rapid decrease in cerebrospinal fluid (CSF) pH (because correction of plasma pH increases pCO_2 both in blood and CSF, but CSF HCO_3 lags behind), leading to the development of neurological manifestations.

Because edema of brain tissue appears to underlie the syndrome, the prevention of a rapid decline in serum osmolarity is effective in preventing DDS. Thus, in the presence of severe uremia, or hypernatremia, the dialysate osmolarity (sodium) should be higher and the difference between dialysate and plasma osmolarity (sodium) should be small. The rate of osmolar change should be slow, which can be achieved by slowing the dialysis process; by using slower Qb and Qd and less efficient dialyzers. In an acute setting, one dialysis session should not attempt to correct the uremic syndrome but, rather, the targeted urea reduction should be less than 30% per treatment during the initial few treatments. Some advocate the use of concurrent dialysate flow to slow the dialytic process in severely uremic patients who are starting dialysis. If the latter is used the dialysate inlet port should still be lower than outlet to prevent issues with the presence of air in the dialysate. Intravenous mannitol solution and the addition of urea to the dialysate have also been used. In severely acidotic patients, dialysate bicarbonate should be reduced for initial dialysis treatments to prevent brain-plasma pH dissociation.

Mild symptoms of DDS (nausea vomiting and headache) are common and are difficult to assign specifically to this syndrome. Treatment is symptomatic. If DDS is suspected, reducing blood and dialysate flow and reducing the UFR slows the dialysis process. Hypertonic solutions can be administered and, if symptoms persist, dialysis treatment should be terminated and the patient managed symptomatically.

In severe cases (obtundation, seizure, or alteration of consciousness), dialysis should be terminated and the symptoms managed medically. Supportive treatment and symptomatic management should be initiated. Intravenous mannitol solution may be useful. With supportive therapy, most patients improve in 24–48 h.

5.1.8.2 Dialyzer-Related Reactions

Adverse reactions are more common with new dialyzers than with reused dialyzers and these adverse reactions are referred to as "first use syndrome." The nonspecific nature of some of these events and the observation that they occur even with reused dialyzers has, however, made this term obsolete. More specifically, most of the events described as a reaction to a dialyzer can be divided into two broad categories—anaphylactic (type A) reactions and nonspecific (type B) reactions.

- Type A reactions: These anaphylactic reactions are typically observed within the first few minutes of dialysis. In their mild form, the patient experiences flushing of the face, itching and urticaria, sneezing, watery eyes, cough, and abdominal cramps or diarrhea. In its severe form, the symptoms include anxiety, a burning sensation at the access site or over the entire body, dyspnea, chest tightness, angioedema, laryngeal edema, respiratory failure, and cardiac arrest, and may result in death. Type A reactions are estimated to occur for about 0.005% of dialyzers sold. In the past, these reactions were seen mainly in patients who were using previously unused hollow fiber dialyzers, as opposed to those using parallel plate versions. Originally, the reactions were considered to be reactions to the cellulosic membrane. The role of ethylene oxide (Eto) was discovered when researchers observed that the majority of patients experiencing these reactions had an IgE antibody specific to the Eto–human serum albumin complex. The potting material of dialyzers is not easily rinsed and is a good store for Eto [10]. It would appear that Eto that had not been rinsed completely out of dialyzers had caused the majority of these reactions; if a good rinsing technique is used, the incidence of type A reactions is lower.

Another set of type A reactions were reported in patients taking angiotensin-converting enzyme (ACE) inhibitors and who were using acrylonitrile (AN)-6 membrane dialyzers [11]. The AN6 membrane would appear to activate Hageman factor, leading to the formation of kallikrein and the subsequent liberation of kinins (including bradykinin). Bradykinin is degraded by ACE and the use of ACE inhibitors increases the circulation of bradykinin, which may produce anaphylactic reactions. It is still unclear whether the membrane or some other factor such as sterilant or dialysate impurity causes these reactions [12], but the role of ACE inhibitors is well documented. There are anecdotal cases of type A reactions with other membranes (such as polyacrylonitrile [PAN] or polysulfone [PS]), but the data with AN6 is the strongest.

Anaphylactic reactions have been reported in patients using high-flux dialyzers and bicarbonate dialysate. Because bicarbonate solution can be contaminated easily, it has been proposed that these contaminants pass across the more permeable membranes, activate the complement cascade, and lead to the allergic reactions.

Reprocessed dialyzers have occasionally been associated with allergic reactions. The possible allergens are contaminated water and sterilizing agents such as formaldehyde or glutaraldehyde. If the rinsing of the dialyzer blood circuit is not carried out properly, the patient may be exposed to formaldehyde. One notable source is the heparin line, especially when improperly clamped and rinsed during the reprocessing of the dialyzer and tubing. Use of ACE inhibitors may augment these reactions.

Other factors that (rarely) may cause allergic reactions include heparin, residual substances from the water filter, and acetate. Isolated reports pointing to each of these have been published. Heparin allergy is not uncommon and should be considered if other agents have been excluded.

Although all of these bradykinin-releasing reactions are exacerbated by ACE inhibitors, angiotensin II antagonists, also known as angiotensin II receptor blockers (ARBs), have no effect on ACE and, in theory, should not be associated with these reactions.

If an anaphylactic reaction is suspected, dialysis must be stopped immediately, blood lines clamped, and blood must not be returned. Further management depends on the severity of symptoms. In mild forms, discontinuation of dialysis and the administration of oxygen and antihistamines may be enough. In more severe cases, steroids, epinephrine, and cardiopulmonary resuscitation may be necessary. Of course, it is best to prevent problems from occurring and the following preventive steps should be carried out:

(i) Dialyzers that have been stored for long periods of time have less Eto-associated problems than dialyzers that arrive fresh from the manufacturer, but a proper Eto rinsing procedure for all dialyzers (and blood tubing) should be used. Use of a sufficient volume of fluid (e.g., 3 l of saline) in the rinsing procedure reduces the risk of a reaction. In Eto-sensitive patients, dialyzers sterilized by other means (e.g., gamma sterilization) should be used. Use of reprocessed dialyzers removes the risk of Eto exposure and even new dialyzers can undergo reuse procedure prior to first use.

(ii) Until the situation is further clarified, patients taking ACE inhibitors should avoid AN6 membrane dialyzers.

(iii) To prevent bacterial contamination, bicarbonate solution should be made in "treated" water (see Section 2.5.2.3 in Chapter 2). Once the solution has been made it must not be allowed to stay unused for long periods (>4 h), because bacteria grow quickly in this medium.

(iv) The dialyzer and blood tubing rinsing procedure should ensure complete removal of all sterilizing agent. All the connecting side branches, such as the heparin line, should be clamped when the dialyzer is rinsed and should be rinsed completely. Failure to do this can cause infusion of sterilant from these branches into the blood (e.g., when heparin is infused).

(v) In sensitive patients heparin can be substituted with citrate or another anticoagulation method can be used.

- Type B reactions: These nonspecific reactions are milder but more common than type A reactions. They typically occur within the first hour of dialysis. The pathogenesis is unclear, but possible factors include activation of the complement by the membrane or by substances found in the dialyzer. These reactions are seen largely with previously unused dialyzers. The main symptoms are chest and back pain. Nasally administered oxygen often helps and dialysis can be continued. Reuse of a dialyzer can be initiated in patients who are prone to these reactions. It is important that coronary artery-related chest pain should be excluded as a possible cause.

5.2 Machine-Related Complications

These accidents are due largely to either mechanical safety system failure or to human failure.

5.2.1 Air Embolism

Manifesting clinically as acute dyspnea, loss of consciousness, seizures, and lower extremity ischemic symptoms, air embolism is an extremely rare (yet life-threatening) complication. With fast blood flow rates ($>300\,\text{ml/min}$), even a small leak has the potential to cause infusion of a large volume of air into the circulatory system. Central venous dialysis catheters are also a source of air embolism. Slow injection of small amounts of air can be handled easily by the circulatory system without any clinical manifestation. However, rapid introduction of a large quantity of air can be lethal.

The position of a patient during dialysis determines the severity of the problem associated with air embolism. If air enters through a peripheral vein (fistula or graft) in a patient sitting upright, it will travel into the cerebral circulation causing cortical damage, convulsions, and coma. Air introduced by a central catheter into the right ventricle can cause acute hypoxia due to a pulmonary air embolism. It can also obstruct the right ventricle and cause a reduction in cardiac output, acute right-sided failure, or severe hypoxia. A patient lying in a head-down (Trendelenburg) position will have lower extremity ischemia because of the movement of the air into the lower extremity veins.

5.2.1.1 Management

Once an air embolism is suspected, dialysis should be stopped immediately and the patient placed on their left side in a head-down position (to trap air at the apex of the right ventricle). This done, endotracheal intubation with oxygen flow at high rate should be started. In severe cases, air may have to aspirated from the right ventricle using a Swan–Ganz catheter.

5.2.2 Hemolysis

Acute hemolysis during dialysis is usually caused by one of the following:

- Oxidizing agents: Chloramine is used as a bacteriostatic agent in municipal water treatment, and is the most common oxidant that causes destruction of erythrocytes during dialysis. Although the charcoal column in the water purification system of the dialysis unit normally removes chloramine, this can fail, causing accidental exposure and widespread hemolysis. Other oxidants that cause hemolysis include copper and nitrates.
- Reducing agents: Formaldehyde is known to cause hemolysis. Exposure occurs when reprocessed dialyzers are rinsed improperly.
- Hyperthermia: Dialysate heated to >45° C, due to failure of the heating system, thermostat, and temperature monitor, can cause massive hemolysis and death.
- Mechanical problems: Pumping blood through a very tight passage can cause severe hemolysis. This occurs when the blood tubing is obstructed and pressure monitoring fails.
- Hypoosmolar dialysate: Failure of the conductivity monitor and proportioning system can lead to the creation of a hypoosmolar dialysate, which can cause hemolysis. Diagnosis of significant hemolysis is not difficult (blood from the dialyzer appears bright red) but chronic and mild hemolysis are difficult to diagnose, unless a diagnostic work-up for hemolysis is undertaken. Treatment includes discontinuation of dialysis; blood in the blood circuit must not be returned. Blood should be obtained for transfusion (typed and cross-matched) and steps should be taken to treat the hyperkalemia that is commonly present.

References

1. De Vries PJ, Kouw PM, van der Meer N et al. Non-invasive monitoring of blood volume during hemodialysis: its relation with post-dialytic dry weight. *Kidney Int* 1993, 44:851–854.
2. Hampl H, Paeprer H, Unger V et al. Hemodynamics during hemodialysis, sequential ultrafiltration and hemofiltration. *J Dial* 1979, 3:51–71.
2a. Pagel MD, Ahmad S, Vizzo JE, Scribner BH: Acetate and bicarbonate fluctuations and acetate intolerance during dialysis. *Kid Int* 1982, 21:513–518.
3. Sadowski RH, Allred EN, Jabs K. Sodium modeling ameliorates intradialytic and interdialytic symptoms in young hemodialysis patients. *Am Soc Nephrol* 1993, 4:1192–1198.
4. Maggiore Q, Pizzarelli F, Zoccali C et al. Influence of blood temperature on vascular stability during hemodialysis and isolated ultrafiltration. *Int J Artif Organs* 1985, 8:175–178.
5. Chazan J. Sudden death in patients with chronic renal failure on hemodialysis. *Dial Transplant* 1987, 16: 447.

6. Amerling R, Cu GA, Dubrow A et al. Complications during hemodialysis. In *Clinical Dialysis, 3rd Edition*. Edited by AR Nissenson, RN Fine, and DE Gentile. Norwalk: Appleton & Lange, 1995; 235–267.

7. Golper TA, Wolfson M, Ahmad S et al. Multicenter trial of l-carnitine in maintenance hemodialysis patients. I. Carnitine concentrations and lipid effects. *Kidney Int* 1990, 38:904–911.

8. Ahmad S, Roberston HT, Golper TA et al. Multicenter trial of l-carnitine in maintenance of hemodialysis patients. II. Clinical and biochemical effects. *Kidney Int* 1990, 38:912–918.

9. Khoss AE, Steger H, Legenstein E et al. L-carnitine therapy and myocardial function in children treated with chronic hemodialysis. *Wien Klin Wochenschr* 1989, 101:17–20.

10. Garnaas KR, Windebank AJ, Blexrud MD et al. Ultrastructure changes produced in dorsal root ganglia in vitro by exposure to ethylene oxide from hemodialysis. *J Neuropathol Exp Neurol* 1991, 50:256–262.

11. Schulman G, Hakim R, Arias R et al. Bradykinin generation by dialysis membranes: possible role in anaphylactic reaction. *Am Soc Nephrol* 1993, 3:1563–1569.

12. Pegues DA, Beck-Sague, Woolen SW et al. Anaphylactoid reactions associated with reuse of hollow-fiber hemodialyzers and ACE inhibitors. *Kidney Int* 1992, 42:1232–1237.

13. Rigby AJ, Scribner BH, Ahmad S. Sodium, not fluid, controls interdialytic weight gain. *Nephrol News & Issues* 2000, 14(9):21–22.

Chapter 6
Dose of Hemodialysis

With the loss of the kidneys, the concentrations of various solutes become abnormal and the total body fluid volume increases. The purpose of dialysis, therefore, is to achieve normalization of solute concentrations and fluid volume. One of the critical roles of dialysis is to reduce the accumulated uremic toxin(s). Unfortunately, measurement of the uremic toxin is not routinely done because we do not have full identification of such a toxin or toxins. We know that urea and creatinine, the commonly used markers for assessing the renal function, are not the uremic toxin. However, today, unfortunately, the dose of dialysis is solely measured and monitored in terms of urea removal. It would be desirable to measure the dose in terms of duration/frequency of treatments, solute removal, as well as fluid control. Blood pressure control and physical assessment of the fluid status should be used for the latter.

6.1 Historical Background

A set of clinical studies by the Seattle group in the late 1960s and early 1970s was the first attempt to define the dose of dialysis [1–3]. From these early studies, three major observations were made:

Duration of dialysis: Adequacy of dialysis was dependent on the duration of dialysis, measured in terms of hours per week.

Dialyzer function: The efficiency of the dialyzer, as determined by the surface area of the membrane, directly influenced the dose of dialysis. Thus, the overall dialysis dose was a function of hours of dialysis per week and the membrane surface area of the dialyzer.

Middle molecule: In the 1960s, it became clear that urea or creatinine were not responsible for uremic syndrome [4, 5]. A set of elegantly designed, prospective, well-controlled studies suggested that a molecule larger than urea (>500 Da) was responsible for uremic neurotoxicity [3]. This molecule was termed middle molecule (MM), because it was larger than small molecules (SM) such as urea and creatinine, and smaller than large molecules such as albumin or peptides. Vi-

S. Ahmad, *Manual of Clinical Dialysis*, DOI 10.1007/978-0-387-09651-3_6,

tamin B_{12} was used as a surrogate marker for this molecule. Because the movement of MM from the extravascular to the vascular compartment is slower than that of SM and it is only removed through the larger pores on the dialyzer membrane that are relatively fewer than are the smaller pores, the total body clearance of MM is more dependent on the duration of dialysis than is the clearance of SM. The clearance of SM is more affected by the speed of dialysis, and blood and dialysate flow rates.

6.1.1 Dialysis Index

Babb et al. [2] proposed a mathematical model to quantify the dose of dialysis using vitamin B_{12} as a surrogate for uremic toxin (MM). The simplified concept of the dialysis index (DI) can be expressed as follows:

$$DImm = \frac{\text{Dialyzer clearance of B12} \times \text{Weekly duration of dialysis (hrs)}}{168 \, hrs \, (= 1 week)}$$

$DImm = K \times t/168$; t = number of hours in one week

If this time-averaged where K = clearance of MM was $30 \, l/week/1.73 \, m^2$ body surface area (BSA) or 2.98 ml/min, the dialysis dose was considered adequate. Significant residual renal function was added to the equation [6], but this complex mathematical model, requiring vitamin B_{12} clearance values, was not widely used in clinical practice.

6.1.2 Urea Clearance

Teschan et al. [7] observed that if patients had a total urea clearance >10 ml/min, they required less blood transfusion and had less uremic problems. They proposed the use of urea clearance relative to its volume of distribution as a means of measuring the dose of dialysis. Thus, a weekly urea clearance of 3,000 ml/week/l of body water (volume of distribution of urea) was considered adequate dialysis. From these studies and from the studies of Gotch et al. [8], the concept of a relationship between dialyzer urea clearance (K), duration of dialysis (t), and volume of distribution of urea (V) was developed. Mathematically, this relationship was designated as dose of dialysis = Kt/V. To calculate this complex, interdependent relationship, a modeling program was devised by Gotch and his colleagues [8], and called urea kinetic modeling (UKM). Initial reports using UKM from the National Co-operative Dialysis Studies suggested that, for a protein intake of >0.8 g/kg/day, a Kt/V value of >0.8 should provide adequate dialysis [9]. Over time, clinical studies have shown that the value of Kt/V should be over 1.2 to prevent under-dialysis and to minimize the consequences of under-dialysis (see Fig. 6.1) [10, 11].

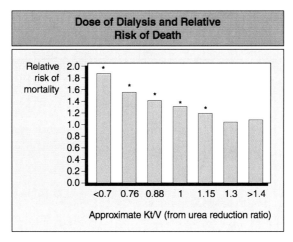

Fig. 6.1 Dose of dialysis and relative risk of death

6.1.3 Urea as a Marker for Uremic Toxins

Although urea itself is not the uremic toxin, it is currently used as a surrogate marker for the uremic toxin, and dialysis dose is quantified in terms of urea removal. The end products of carbohydrate and fat metabolism are removed by the lungs and by the skin, whereas the waste products of protein metabolism are removed by the kidneys. Therefore, it is logical to assume that uremic symptoms must be caused by the accumulation of the products of protein metabolism. Because urea is also a product of protein metabolism, it seems reasonable to use it as the marker for uremic toxin(s). Urea is, however, a small (molecular weight 60 Da), electrically neutral molecule and is thus capable of moving easily across various body compartments. For this reason, its dialytic clearance is more dependent on the rate of removal than on the duration of dialysis. If the uremic toxin is larger than urea, is electrically charged, and/or has a rate of flux across cell membranes that differs from that of urea, kinetic behavior during dialysis will be different from that of urea and urea would not be a good marker. The major advantages of using urea as the marker are that it is easily measured, that it is tested routinely, and that its metabolism, generation rate, and volume of distribution are well known. In addition, urea can be used to estimate protein intake.

6.1.4 Current Methods of Measuring Dialysis Dose

The current techniques for the measurement of dialysis dose are based on the removal of urea by dialysis. There are three methods commonly used, each with a different degree of difficulty and accuracy.

6.1.4.1 Urea Reduction Ratio

The percentage decline in urea concentration during a dialysis session is a direct result of that treatment. The magnitude of decline can therefore be used to measure the dose of dialysis.

The efficacy of dialysis in terms of urea removal is dependent on the urea clearance capacity of the dialyzer, the blood and dialysate flow, and to a lesser degree the duration of dialysis. The easiest method of dose determination is to measure both the predialysis and postdialysis blood urea nitrogen (BUN) concentrations and to calculate the percent reduction (urea reduction rate [URR]).

$$\text{URR} = \{1 - [\text{postdialysis BUN concentration (post-BUN)}/\text{predialysis BUN}$$
$$\text{concentration (pre-BUN)}]\} \times 100$$

Example

$$\text{Pre-BUN} = 90\,\text{mg/dl}; \text{post-BUN} = 25\,\text{mg/dl}; \text{thus}, \text{URR} = [1 - (25/90)]$$
$$\times 100 = 72\%$$

Currently, a URR of 65% (equivalent to a Kt/V of 1.2) is considered to be the minimum acceptable level for adequate dialysis.

6.1.4.2 Calculating Kt/V from Urea Reduction

Kt/V can be calculated using urea reduction, ultrafiltered volume, and dialysis duration. Several reasonably accurate formulae calculate Kt/V from these (see below).

Simple linear formula:

$$\text{Kt/V} = 2.2 - \{3.3 \times [\text{R} - (0.03 - \text{UF/W})]\},$$

where $\text{R} = \text{post-BUN/pre-BUN}; \text{UF} = \text{predialysis weight} - \text{postdialysis weight};$ and $\text{W} = \text{postdialysis weight}$. This formula assumes a linear relationship between R and Kt/V, which is not precise. The Kt/V can, however, be calculated easily. Thus, in the example discussed above, if the patient loses 2 kg of weight and the postdialysis weight is 70 kg, the $\text{Kt/V} = 2.2 - \{3.3 \times [0.27 - (0.032/70)]\} = 1.50$. This formula provides a rough estimate but is not very accurate or reliable.

Logarithmic formulae:

Because the relationship between Kt/V and URR is more logarithmic than linear, two logarithmic formulae provide accurate and reproducible results:

$$1.\ \text{Kt/V} = \frac{-\ln \text{R} + (3 \times [\text{UF/W}])}{1 - 0.01786\,t}$$

2. $Kt/V = [-\ln (R - 0.008 \times t)] + [(4 - 3.5 \times R) \times (UF/W)][12]$

where $\ln$ = natural log and t = the duration of dialysis in hours.

Example

Using the above formulae, if the patient dialyzes for 3 h: Formula 1 yields $Kt/V = \{(\ln 0.27) + [3(2/70)]\}/[1(0.017863)] = 1.47$; and Formula 2 yields $Kt/V = \{[\ln 0.27(0.0083)]\} + \{[4(3.50.27)]\}(2/70) = 1.41$.

6.1.4.3 Urea Kinetic Modeling

Computerized programs can calculate Kt/V using complex formulae that are based on the interrelationship of dialyzer clearance, urea decline, and the volume of distribution of urea. The basic steps are as follows:

1. Input the in vitro dialyzer urea clearance (K) value from the manufacturer's sheet (for the appropriate blood flow rate). From this, the program estimates the in vivo clearance value, or uses the dialyzer clearance value from the mass transfer coefficient (KoA).
2. Input the pre-BUN and post-BUN, weight values, and duration of dialysis (t). From this, the program calculates a delivered Kt/V value. It then computes a modeled value for the volume of distribution (V) of urea from the estimated K, t, and the slope of the intradialytic urea decline curve (see Fig. 6.2).

The modeled V is then compared with the V value derived from the nomogram to identify treatment-related problems.

6.2 Potential Problems with the Calculation of Dialysis Dose

Even if the issue of using urea as the surrogate marker for the uremic toxin is omitted, other problems with the current methods of calculating dialysis dose exist. The most significant source of error is based on the assumption that urea movement is so rapid that it can be considered to be distributed in a single pool in the body.

6.2.1 Influence of the Single-Pool Model

Urea does not always behave as a solute distributed in a single pool. When dialysis ceases, the rate of blood urea increase is not linear; there may be at least two different phases, with a very steep initial curve followed by a less steep curve (see Fig. 6.2).

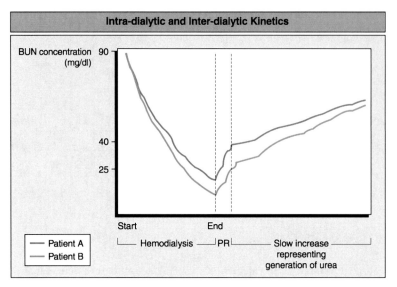

Fig. 6.2 Plots **A** and **B** represent two patients undergoing the same treatment (blood flow rate, dialysate flow rate, and ultrafiltration rate). The difference in the slope can be used to determine the volume of distribution (V) and generation rate. Thus, patient A has a larger V-value than patient B has, for urea. *BUN* blood urea nitrogen, *PR* postdialysis rebound

In the example shown in Fig. 6.2, the BUN concentration drops, for patient A, from 90 to 25 mg/dl during a single dialysis session, giving a URR of 72%, but when the measurement is repeated 30 min later, the BUN has increased to 40 mg/dl—a rise that reflects the movement of urea from the extravascular to the vascular space; the steadily increasing curve following this initial steep rise represents the generation of urea. This means that the overall impact of dialysis was equivalent to a urea reduction of 55% (not 72%, an approximate Kt/V of 1.0 not 1.3).

The behavior of urea in this example is that of a solute distributed in more than one pool. It should be clear from this that the timing of blood sampling for urea determination is critical in obtaining the correct URR value and the delivered dose of dialysis. Several factors, such as speed of dialysis, recirculation (peripheral and cardiopulmonary) of dialyzed blood, and poor perfusion of blood to tissue with a larger amount of urea, influence the equilibration between vascular and extravascular spaces or slope of curve. The fact that the dialyzer, attached to arteriovenous (AV) access, can be viewed as being connected in parallel to the rest of the body influences the efficiency of urea removal from the whole body. Thus, very efficient removal of urea (ultra-efficient dialysis) will deplete the vascular spaces of urea at a faster rate than the rest of the body, leading to a very steep decline in BUN. As soon as dialysis is stopped, however, a fast equilibration rapidly increases the BUN.

6.2.1.1 Correcting for the Two-Pool Model

Because it is not practical to wait 30 min to obtain each postdialysis urea sample, two methods of correction for the two-pool model are available. Postdialysis urea rebound can be measured by obtaining blood samples both immediately after and 30 min after the cessation of dialysis, and a correction factor determined from these data. This correction factor can be applied for future values, although, for accuracy, the rebound should be measured more than once. Because the rebound is influenced by the duration and rate of dialysis and by body size, mathematical formulae are available to correct for this effect. Under similar circumstances, the rebound is less marked ($<30\%$) with venous central access (catheter) than with AV access. The two formulae for obtaining calculated equilibrated Kt/V (eKt/V) from the unequilibrated single-pool Kt/V are:

For AV access: $eKt/V = Kt/V - \{0.6 \times [(Kt/V)/t]\} + 0.03$
For central venous catheters: $eKt/V = Kt/V - \{0.4 \times [(Kt/V)/t]\} + 0.02$

where Kt/V is obtained by using the immediate post-BUN from either the arteriovenous or venous access.

6.2.1.2 Urea Kinetic Modeling

Although this is a very reproducible method of determining the Kt/V, it does have several potential sources of error. Some of these have been addressed, but readers should be aware of the potential pitfalls, because the method is computerized, complex, and not easily understood.

Access recirculation: In instances of access recirculation, the actual K will be lower than that used in the formula. Consequently, the actual delivered Kt/V will be lower than the calculated value.

Dialyzer clearance: Accurate determination of K is a problem, and using the in vitro value that the manufacturer provides (which is usually an overestimate) leads to overestimation of Kt/V.

Effect of dialysate, blood flow rates, and clotted fibers: Each of these influences the actual K value and, as such, the delivered Kt/V will again be lower than anticipated.

Time of dialysis: Any mistake in actual dialysis time compared with expected dialysis time will influence the results. If alarm interruptions, for example, are not factored in, the actual t will be shorter than the prescribed t, this will overestimate the Kt/V.

Volume of distribution problems: Determination of V from the slope of the curve can be problematic, depending on the timing of the postdialysis blood sampling. Thus, while a steeper curve, based on a blood sample taken immediately after dialysis, may suggest a smaller volume of distribution, a 30-min wait may show a less steep decline and a larger actual volume of distribution (see Fig. 6.3).

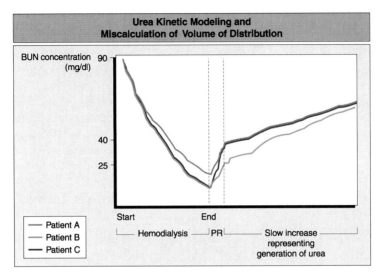

Fig. 6.3 For **A** and **B**, refer to Fig. 6.2. In this example, a third patient **C** Behaves like **B**, but has a steeper rebound. If rebound was not measured, this patient would be considered to have a volume of distribution (V) for urea smaller than the actual value of V, thus leading to miscalculation of dose of dialysis (Kt/V). *BUN* blood urea nitrogen, *PR* postdialysis rebound

To minimize the impact of these problems, the procedure used must follow the recommended steps and verification guidelines strictly.

6.2.1.3 Residual Renal Function

When dialysis is first initiated, some patients may have residual renal function (K_{ru}) that is sufficient to have a significant impact on total uremic control; lowering the treatment requirement. However, it is not advisable to reduce treatment time based on renal function without frequent measurement of this function because it may decline rapidly, increasing the risk of under-dialysis. The potential errors in the measurement of K_{ru} and its impact on the dose of dialysis should also be considered.

When postdialysis blood is collected for urea measurement, the patient must empty their bladder (the urine is discarded). From this time, all urine must be collected and brought to the dialysis unit when the patient returns for the next dialysis. Again, the patient should be asked to void urine and collect that volume in a container. Predialysis blood should be collected for urea measurement, the time between the two dialyses noted, and K_{ru} calculated as follows:

Urine urea concentration (mg/dl) urine volume (ml)
K_{ru} = Urine urea concentration (mg/dl) × urine volume (ml)/([post BUN + pre − BUN]/2(mg/dl) × time between dialysis (minutes)

Example

Post-BUN $= 20 \, mg/dl$ (collected at 11:00 Monday)
Next Pre-BUN $= 80 \, mg/dl$ (collected at 07:00 Wednesday)
Urine volume $= 1.5L$; urine urea nitrogen $= 200 \, mg/dl$

$$K_{ru} = 200 \, mg/dl \times 1500 \, ml/[(20 \, mg/dl + 80 \, mg/dl/2)] \times (44 \times 60) \text{minutes}$$
$$= 2.27 \, ml/min$$

Once K_{ru} is calculated, it can be used to calculate total Kt/V, using the following formula (devised by Gotch):

For a patient dialyzing three times a week, the total combined $KT/V = (Kt/V) + [5.5 \times (K_{ru}/V)]$. For a patient dialyzing twice a week, the total combined $KT/V = (Kt/V) + (9.5 \times (K_{ru}/V))$, where V = volume of distribution of urea (V can be calculated from BSA).

Measuring residual renal function in hemodialysis (HD): The reasons for the measurement of K_{ru} in HD are listed in Table 6.1; it is not advisable to use this value to reduce the time of dialysis unless the measurements are repeated monthly so that an unexpected decline would lead to an increase in dialysis time and risk of under-dialysis can be avoided. Recognizing this, the new Dialysis Outcome Quality Initiative (DOQI) guideline does not recommend routine measurement of K_{ru} (Table 6.2).

Table 6.1 Reasons to Measure residual renal function in hemodialysis

1. To measure total toxin removal:
   - To calculate T, dialyze just long enough to get minimum $Kt/V_{urea} \to 1.2$
     - Risk of under-dialysis for MM
     - Risk of persistent extracellular volume excess and hypertension
2. To calculate DPI from nPCR (nPNA):
   Urea generated between two dialyses comes from protein catabolism that is equal to protein intake (this relationship is controversial)
3. To predict outcome:
   - Its value to predict outcome is unclear

Table 6.2 New KDOQI recommendation ("stop" and "cap")

Frequency	Minimum (target) SpKt/V	
	$K_{ru} < 2$	$K_{ru} > 2$
Two per week	Not recommended	2.0 (2.3)
Three per week	1.2 (1.4)	0.9 (1.15)
Four per week	0.8 (0.9)	0.6 (0.7)

$K_{ru} < 2.0 \, ml/min/1.73 \, m^2 \to$ No reduction in Kt/V target (1.4, 15% higher than minimum of 1.2)
$K_{ru} > 2.0 \, ml/min$, reduce minimum Kt/V by 20%

6.2.1.4 Normalized Protein Catabolic Rate

In stable patients who are neither catabolic nor anabolic, the dietary protein intake (DPI) correlates tightly with the protein catabolic rate (PCR), and the urea generation rate correlates well with the PCR. Thus, from the postdialysis and predialysis urea measurements and the changes in volume of distribution of urea (total body water [TBW]), the urea generation rate and thus both PCR and DPI can be calculated. This relationship has been found experimentally to be:

$$\text{Urea generation rate (g/day)} = [0.154 \times \text{PCR(g/day)}] - 1.7$$

In the National Cooperative Dialysis Study (NCDS) a reduced rate of morbidity was observed in patients with high normalized PCR (nPCR) [9], presumably reflecting a higher DPI. Studies have shown a beneficial effect of good PCR (DPI) and serum albumin on survival of patients [11]. Thus, it is important to estimate nPCR as a part of dialysis dose measurement. UKM uses the rate of increase in BUN between dialysis sessions to calculate nPCR. In those patients with a significant urine output, it is important to include loss of nitrogen in urine. Formulae (see below) or nomograms (see Fig. 6.4) can be used to estimate nPCR from a mid-week pre-BUN and post-BUN.

$$\text{nPCR} = 0.0186 \, (1 - 0.162 \, \text{R})(1 - [\text{R} + \text{UF}/\text{V}])\text{Cpre}/1 - 0.0003 \, \text{t}$$

where nPCR = normalized PCR, V = volume of distribution of urea (either determined from Watson's formula [see Section 9.21] or taken to be $0.58 \times$ dry weight), Cpre = predialysis BUN, and t = dialysis time in minutes.

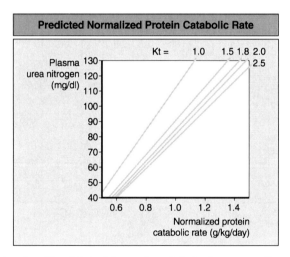

Fig. 6.4 Values based on Kt and first-of-the week predialysis plasma urea nitrogen (after the long interdialytic interval) in patients dialyzed twice weekly. Kt urea clearance rate (reproduced with permission from [13])

This formula ignores, however, the effect of timing of blood sampling. BUN prior to the first dialysis of the week is higher than that obtained prior to the second or third dialysis of the week. Pre-BUN is expected to be lowest for the third dialysis of the week. The following formulae have been proposed to take these variations into account and enable PCR (the term protein equivalent of nitrogen appearance rate [PNA] is preferred by some) to be calculated more accurately:

For the first dialysis of the week:

$$PCR \ (PNA) = (C_o/[36.3 + 5.48 \times Kt/V + 53.5/Kt/V]) + 0.168$$

For the second dialysis of the week:

$$PCR \ (PNA) = (C_o/[25.8 + 1.15 \times Kt/V + 56.4/Kt/V]) + 0.168$$

For the last dialysis of the week:

$$PCR \ (PNA) = (C_o/[16.3 + 4.30 \times Kt/V + 56.6/Kt/V]) + 0.168$$

In patients with significant residual renal function, the adjusted PCR (PNA) is calculated by substituting $C_{o/}$ with $C_r = C_o \times (1 + [0.79 + 3.08/Kt/VKr/V])$, where C_o = pre-BUN (mg/dl); Kt/V = single pool Kt/V; Kr/V = residual urinary urea clearance (ml/min); and V = volume of disturbance of urea (14)

Recent data have raised questions about the value of calculating nPCR for the following reasons:

1. The nPCR (DPI) have not been shown to predict outcome
2. The calculation of DPI from nPCR may not be accurate

Frequency of dialysis and Standard Kt/V (StdKt/V) concept: The discussion of dose measurement so far has centered around three times a week dialysis. Over the last decade, more frequent dialysis has gained popularity. Frequent dialysis requires a different concept of dose calculation. As seen in Fig. 6.5, more frequent dialysis is associated with lower peak urea concentration, and a lower Kt/V value is needed for each dialysis to achieve same results as a Kt/V of 1.2 for three times a week dialysis. To calculate the comparable Kt/V values for different frequencies (2–7 HD), the concept of standard Kt/V (StdKt/V) has been developed. This is based on the concept of urea clearance equivalent to renal clearance or eK_{ru} and is applicable to varying frequencies of HD, PD and continuous therapies.

eK_{ru}: In steady state, the urea clearance by the kidney should be equal to the amount of urea removed divided by the plasma urea concentration:

$$Urea \ clearance = (urine \ urea \times urine \ volume) \div plasma \ urea$$

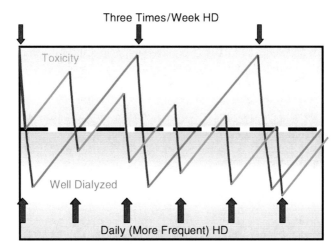

Fig. 6.5 Pre and post dialysis urea concentration (Y axis) with three times and more frequent dialysis (arrows). Area above the dashed line represents toxic (underdialyis) concentrations and below line well dialyzed levels of urea. With more frequent treatments the required urea reduction per treatment (URR or Kt/V) to achieve good dialysis is less than with less frequent dialyses

Let us take a hypothetical case in which a patient is continuously dialyzed for 1 week. The urea clearance in this patient would be similar to the urea clearance by a natural kidney. Now let us assume the patient is getting 6 days of dialysis and each session lasts 2 h. In this patient, the dialysis urea clearance equivalent to renal urea clearance (eK_{ru}) would be urea generation (G) divided by time average concentration (TAC) of urea (similar to UV/P). The G can be calculated from postdialysis and the next predialysis urea concentrations and the TAC from several predialysis BUN measurements. Thus K = G/mean urea concentration. The mean urea concentration can be calculated from several predialysis urea measurements (see below).

Example

A 70-kg patient dialyzes for 2 h, 6 days a week. His g = 8 g/day; and his BUNs measured three times (Monday, Wednesday, and Friday) are 60, 55, and 54, respectively; thus, his mean (TAC) urea is $(60 + 55 + 54)/3 = 55$ mg/dl. The TBW is 55% of body weight, or 38.5 l (volume of distribution of urea or V).

$$G = 8\,g/24\,h \text{ or } 5.6\,mg/min \text{ per } 38.5\,L$$
$$eK_{ru} = 5.6\,mg/min \div 55\,mg/100\,ml$$
$$= 10.2\,ml/min \text{ or } 10.2 \times 1,008\,min/week = 10.2\,L/week$$

StdKt/V: StdKt/V is a method where a one week K (for all the treatments over one week) is normalized to the V (volume of distribution of urea). At least two formulae are available to calculate this, Gotch's and Leypoldt's formulae.

Gotch's formula:

$$\text{StdKt/V} = \frac{0.184(\text{nPCR} - 1.17) \times V \times 0.001}{\text{Mean urea concentration}} \times \frac{7 \times 1440}{V}$$

First part of the formula is G, thus formula can be written as:

$$\text{StdKt/V} = \frac{G(\text{mg/min})}{\text{Mean urea concentration}} \times \frac{10080}{V}$$

Leypoldt formula can be used for intermittent as well as continuous therapies:

$$\text{StdKt/V} = \frac{168 \times (1 - \exp[-\text{eqKt/V}])/t/60}{[(1 - \exp(-\text{eqKt/V}))/\text{eq}/\text{Kt/V} + 168/N/(t/60) - 1]}$$

Where N = number of treatments per week
And, $\text{eqKt/V} = 0.924 \times \text{spKt/V} - 0.395 \times \text{spKt/V}/(t/60) + 0.056$

Leypoldt's formula can also be written as:

$$\text{StdKt/V} = \frac{1008 \frac{1 - e^{-\text{eKt/V}}}{t}}{\frac{1 - -\text{eKt/V}}{\text{spKt/V}} + \frac{1008}{Nt - 1}}$$

where t is the dialysis session duration in minutes and N is number of dialysis treatments per week.

   The StdKt/V of 2.0 is considered the minimum adequate dose of dialysis for all treatment modalities.

6.3 Determining Adequate Dialysis

Unfortunately, each of the studies looking at the adequacy of dialysis dose has been designed in such a way that the dose identified is that below which there is increased morbidity and mortality (the minimum dose). Questions now need to be asked about the optimum dialysis, a dose which, if increased further, is not associated with any further improvement in morbidity or mortality statistics (the optimum dose).

   Further, the dose has, to date, been defined only in terms of solute clearance, and the issue of volume (fluid) control, another critical function of dialysis, has not been addressed adequately. It is clear that control of hypertension in the dialysis patient has a direct impact on survival and that appropriate fluid volume control leads to adequate blood pressure control. Fluid volume control is easier with longer dialysis than with shorter dialysis, but it is unclear whether this is secondary to better volume control or the better MM clearance that is observed with longer dialysis.

The best survival for dialysis patients has been reported by Charra et al. [15] and it is worth noting that their patients were dialyzed for longer than usual (very good MM clearance) and that <5% of their patients required blood pressure medications. This suggests that future work should focus on the impact of MM clearance and volume control as critical components of the measurement of dose of dialysis.

6.3.1 Acceptable Kt/V Values

In general, it is now accepted that the minimum Kt/V value of >0.9 defined by NCDS is inadequate, with most people accepting the National Kidney Foundation (NKF)-DOQI guidelines value of 1.2 (some consider 1.4 the acceptable minimum value). It is important to remember that if post-BUN is measured immediately after dialysis and Kt/V is determined to be 1.3, the equilibrated Kt/V may be as low as 1.0 if the patient has a large postdialysis urea rebound. The more uniformly useable concept of StdKt/V suggests that the minimum acceptable dose should be 2.0.

6.3.2 Frequency of Dose Measurement

At present, the practice of measuring the dose once a quarter or once a month may be too infrequent. Recently, it was observed that Kt/V correlates well with the volume of blood dialyzed [16]. This value is available for each dialysis and can be used to monitor the dose for every treatment. The effect of the volume of blood dialyzed on patient outcome has, however, not been studied.

References

1. Babb AL, Popovich RP, Christopher TG et al. The genesis of square meter-hour hypothesis. *Trans Am Soc Artif Intern Organs* 1971, 17:81–91.
2. Babb AL, Strand MD, Uvelli DA et al. Quantitive description of dialysis treatment: a dialysis index. *Kidney Int* 1975, 2:23–29.
3. Scribner BH. Discussion. *Trans Am Soc Artif Intern Organs* 1965, 11:29.4; Johnson WJ, Hagge WW, Wagoner RD et al. Effects of urea loading in patients with far-advanced renal failure. *Mayo Clin Proc* 1972, 47:21–29.
4. Milutinovic J, Babb AL, Eschbach JW et al. Uremic neuropathy: evidence of middle molecule toxicity. *Artif Organs* 1978, 2:45–51.
5. Ahmad S, Babb AL, Milutinovic J et al. Effect of residual renal function on minimum dialysis requirements. *Proc Eur Dial Transplant Assoc* 1979, 16:107–114.
6. Teschan PE, Ginn HE, Bourne, JR et al. Neurobehavioral probes for adequacy of dialysis. *Trans Am Soc Artif Intern Organs* 1977, 23:556–559.
7. Gotch FA. A quantitative evaluation of small molecule and middle molecule toxicity in therapy of uremia. *Dial Transplant* 1980, 9:183–186.

8. Gotch F, Sargent J. A mechanistic analysis of the National Cooperative Dialysis Study (NCDS). *Kidney Int* 1985, 28:526–534.
9. Garred LJ, Canaud BC, McCready WG. Optimal hemodialysis—The role of quantification. *Sem Dial* 1994, 7:236–240.
10. Owen WF Jr, Lew NL, Liu Y et al. The urea reduction ratio and serum albumin concentrations as predictors of mortality in patients undergoing hemodialysis. *N Engl J Med* 1993, 329:1001–1006.
11. Daugirdas JT. Simplified equations for monitoring Kt/V, PCRn, eKt/V and ePRCn. *Adv Ren Replace Ther* 1995, 2:295–304.
12. Daugirdas JT. Estimation of equilibrated Kt/V using unequilibrated postdialysis BUN. *Sem Dial* 1995, 8:23–26.
13. Daugirdas JT, Depner TA. A nomogram approach to hemodialysis urea modeling. *Am J Kidney Dis* 1994, 23:33–40.
14. Depner T, Daugirdas J. Equations for normalized protein catabolic rate based on two-point modeling of hemodialysis urea kinetics. *J Am Soc Nepherol* 1996 7:780–785.
15. Charra B, Calemard E, Cuche M, et al. Control of hypertension and prolonged survival on maintenance hemodialysis. *Nephrol* 1983, 33:96–102.
16. Ahmad S. A simple method to monitor the dose of hemodialysis. *ASAIO J* 1997, 43:298–302.

Chapter 7
Continuous Therapies

Robert M Winrow, MD
Suhail Ahmad, MD

7.1 Overview

Critically ill patients with acute kidney injury can be too unstable to tolerate conventional intermittent dialysis therapies (IHD). With continuous therapies, the rate of fluid removal and solute exchange is decreased thus leading to improved patient tolerance of the procedure. Continuous renal replacement therapies (CRRT) take advantage of two methods of fluid and solute removal: diffusion-based solute removal (dialysis), or convection-based solute and fluid removal (filtration), or both simultaneously. The reported benefits of CRRT therapy in critically ill patients include:

– Less hemodynamic instability
– Better tolerance to ultrafiltration
– Removal of immunomodulatory substances with convective therapies
– Less effect on intracranial pressure

7.2 Types of Continuous Therapies

– Continuous arteriovenous hemofiltration (CAVH)
– Continuous venovenous hemofiltration (CVVH)
– Continuous venovenous hemodialysis (CVVHD)
– Continuous venovenous hemodiafiltration (CVVHDF)
– Slow low-efficiency diffusion hemodialysis (SLEDD)
– Slow continuous ultrafiltration (SCUF) See Table 7.1

7.2.1 Continuous Arteriovenous Hemofiltration (CAVH)

The initial description of the CAVH technique by Kramer in 1977 [1] used blood drawn directly from an artery, passed into a hemofilter, and returned to a vein. The

S. Ahmad, *Manual of Clinical Dialysis*, DOI 10.1007/978-0-387-09651-3_7,
© Springer Science+Business Media LLC 2009

Table 7.1 Comparison of techniques [12]

	IHD	CVVH	CVVHD	CVVHDF	SLEDD	SCUF
Membrane permeability	Variable	High	High	High	Variable	High
Blood flow rate (ml/min)	250–400	200–300	100–300	200–300	100–200	100–200
Dialysate flow rate (ml/min)	500–800	0	16–35	16–35	100–300	0
Filtrate (l/day)	0–4	24–96	0–4	24–48	0–24	0–24
Replacement fluid (l/day)	0	21–90	0	23–44	0	0
Effluent saturation (urea, %)	15–40	100	85–100	85–100	60–70	100
Solute clearance	Diffusion	Convection	Diffusion	Diffusion + convection	Diffusion	Convection (minimal)
Urea clearance (ml/min)	180–240	17–67	22	30–60	75–90	1.7
Duration (h)	3–6	> 24	> 24	> 24	Variable	Variable

systemic arterial pressure drove the system without a blood pump, similar to earlier dialysis using Scribner's shunt. Ultrafiltration at a slower rate was controlled by gravitational force, by varying the height of the collection bag from the patient. The ultrafiltrate was replaced by a fluid similar in composition to dialysate. If the replacement fluid was added prior to the hemofilter, the technique was called pre-dilution, whereas fluid replacement after the filter was called post-dilution (see Fig. 7.1).

Thus, CAVH had the following potential advantages:

- No machines, pumps, monitors, or specially trained staff required
- Hemodynamic stability due to slow convective clearance
- Easier management of volume load
- Theoretically improved middle molecule clearance compared with diffusion dialysis

7.2.2 Continuous Venovenous Hemofiltration (CVVH)

Although CAVH had the above advantages, the system still required arterial access, with associated complication rates in the 3–28% range [2, 3]. These complications included arteriovenous fistula, arterial embolization, pseudoaneurysm, arterial

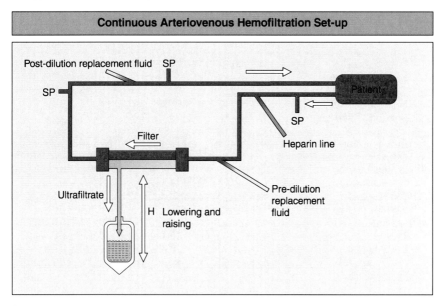

Fig. 7.1 *SP* sampling port, *H* height of collection bag

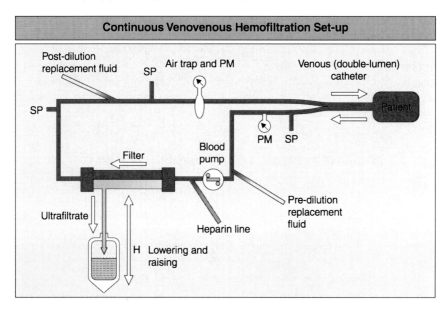

Fig. 7.2 *SP* sampling port; *PM* pressure monitor, *H* height of the collection bag

hemorrhage, and infection. Subsequently, venous access came to dominate CRRT vascular access. This required the addition of a blood pump with associated power, monitors, and technology similar to that of IHD, except that the dialysate circuit was not required (see Fig. 7.2). Table 7.2 shows the ratio between the concentration

Table 7.2 Relation of ultrafiltrate to plasma with CAVH

	Ultrafiltrate (UF)	Plasma (P)	UF/P ratio
Sodium (mEq/l)	135.3 ± 11.2	136.2 ± 10.37	0.993 ± 0.023
Potassium (mEq/l)	4.05 ± 0.71	4.11 ± 0.66	0.985 ± 0.055
Chloride (mEq/l)	103.7 ± 9.55	99.3 ± 10.8	1.046 ± 0.037
Bicarbonate (mEq/l)	22.13 ± 5.08	19.78 ± 4.69	1.124 ± 0.085
Blood urea nitrogen (mg/dl)	82.9 ± 38.4	79.1 ± 36.1	1.048 ± 0.024
Creatinine (mg/dl)	6.63 ± 4.00	6.5 ± 3.86	1.020 ± 0.074
Uric acid (mg/dl)	7.54 ± 3.33	7.35 ± 3.00	1.016 ± 0.081
Phosphorus (mg/dl)	4.15 ± 1.29	3.94 ± 1.13	1.044 ± 0.078
Glucose (mg/dl)	173 ± 84.5	164.5 ± 76.6	1.043 ± 0.055
Total proteins (g/dl)	0.13 ± 0.13	6.21 ± 0.32	0.021 ± 0.021
Albumin (g/dl)	0.02 ± 0.04	2.65 ± 0.46	0.008 ± 0.016
Calcium (mg/dl)	5.12 ± 0.42	8.08 ± 0.61	0.637 ± 0.071
Total bilirubin (mg/dl)	0.44 ± 0.55	12.1 ± 9.52	0.030 ± 0.029
Direct bilirubin (mg/dl)	0.26 ± 0.31	7.35 ± 5.89	0.030 ± 0.019
Creatinine phosphokinase (IU)	66.5 ± 88.3	80.9 ± 88.2	0.676 ± 0.215

All values are expressed as means ± standard deviation. N = 10 samples. Reproduced from [4] with permission

of common plasma constituents in the ultrafiltrate and plasma [4]. If the ratio of ultrafiltrate to plasma (sieving coefficient) is 1, then the clearance of that solute is equal to the ultrafiltration rate. Volume removed/replaced was often not enough to achieve sufficient solute removal (dialysis) and risk of under-dialysis became an issue, particularly in catabolic adult patients.

7.2.3 Continuous Venovenous Hemodialysis (CVVHD)

In CVVHD, dialysate is run through the membrane in a slow continuous manner. Diffusion is the primary method of solute removal and the total amount of fluid is significantly lower than in CVVH, because this equals the volume to be removed to control volume overload. Although there is convective clearance with this fluid removal, it is a relatively small addition to the diffusive clearance.

With the transition to venovenous access in the mid 1980s [5], the dialysis machine became both more complicated and more accurate. The pump-driven venovenous circuit allowed for more precision and higher blood flow rates as compared with the arterial pressure-driven CAVH circuits. However, the use of the blood pump also necessitated safety systems to monitor for venous air embolus, air detectors with occlusion clamps, and the use of pressure transducers. An additional benefit was that large-bore arterial access was no longer needed.

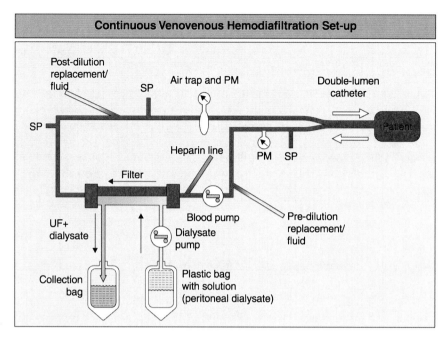

Fig. 7.3 *SP* sampling port, *PM* pressure monitor

7.2.4 Continuous Venovenous Hemodiafiltration (CVVHDF)

The convective clearance of CVVH is not always sufficient to maintain adequate solute clearance in extremely catabolic critically ill patients. Therefore, solute removal was increased by allowing dialysate to flow at a slow rate across the filter, thus adding diffusive to convective clearance. This continuous combined hemofiltration and dialysis was called continuous hemodiafiltration (CAVHDF or CVVHDF, depending on the blood access, Fig. 7.3). To prevent contamination across the permeable hemofilters, sterile pyrogen-free dialysate (such as peritoneal dialysate) was used. The system still did not require the dialysate-related technological complexities of the usual hemodialysis (HD) machines. The continuous slower speed of treatment was still better tolerated than intermittent treatments.

7.2.5 Slow Low-Efficiency Diffusion Hemodialysis (SLEDD)

Current CVVHDF therapies take advantage of integrated systems to successfully offer this therapy (see Section 7.3.6 Machines, below). However, the systems have a number of drawbacks, including:

– Initial cost of the specialized CRRT machines
– Component costs (tubing, dialyzers) customized for the CRRT machine

- Nursing training for the CRRT machines
- Replacement fluid logistics and costs
- Increased patient care complexity for intensive care nurses managing CRRT machines

Thus, interest developed in using regular hemodialysis machines (used for intermittent therapy) to offer continuous renal replacement support. SLEDD therapies slow down the solute removal rate by decreasing both blood and dialysate flows for continuous use. By using conventional IHD machines and adjusting blood flows into the 100–200 ml/min range and dialysate flows to 100–300 ml/min, it is possible to offer CRRT with these machines, and the treatment is better tolerated with relatively more overall solute removal. The cost is also lower because special dialysate and replacement fluids are not required.

7.2.6 Slow Continuous Ultrafiltration (SCUF)

SCUF is used mainly to control fluid excess without a diffusive process, thus, it is hemodynamically better tolerated. However, the overall solute removal by this convective process is much lower than with hemofiltration because the UF volume is relatively small. With continuous therapy, up to 15+ l of fluid per day can be removed.

7.2.7 Newer Technologies

With the increasing interest in SLEDD for CRRT, and to provide additional convective transport by hemofiltration or hemodiafiltration that would be less complex and expensive, "online" generation of replacement fluid for the SLEDD machines has been developed. Thus, the ability of IHD machines to generate large quantities of less expensive dialysate (up to 800 ml/min) is tapped. To have the fluid generated from the dialysate free of contaminants, an extra set of filters is inserted (see Fig. 7.4).

With the ability to generate large volumes of replacement fluids quickly and easily, SLEDD therapy with online hemodiafiltration will become another option for CRRT therapies offering combined convective and diffusive clearance.

Another variation on hemodiafiltration with SLEDD therapy is the concept of "mid-dilution hemofiltration." A specially designed hemofilter has an inner and outer compartment, with blood entering on the side of the header, and traveling down the outer section. At the other end of the membrane, replacement fluid is infused, it mixes with the blood and travels back down the central component of the membrane to exit centrally (see Fig. 7.5).

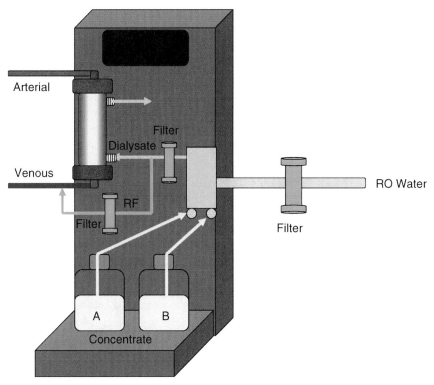

Fig. 7.4 On-line hemodiafiltration set up, generation of RF from dialysate. 3-barrier filtration system. RO = reverse osmosis unit; RF = Replacement fluid

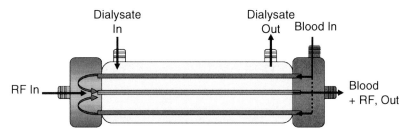

Fig. 7.5 Mid-dilution Hemofilter

Nephros, Inc. (New York, NY), founded by members of Columbia University, has developed a proprietary system that uses the mid-dilution concept along with online replacement fluid generation to offer hemodiafiltration with a conventional dialysis machine. The system is currently undergoing clinical trials, and may offer another option for CRRT therapies in the near future (see Fig. 7.6).

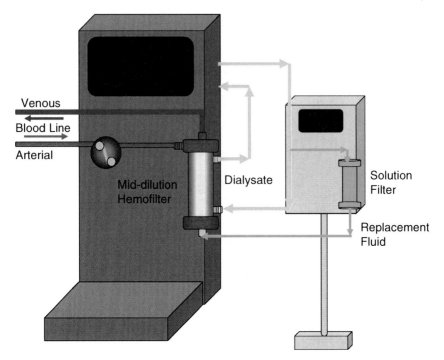

Fig. 7.6 Mid-dilution hemofiltration system with on-line fluid generation

7.3 Components of Continuous Therapies

7.3.1 Vascular Access

The CAVH and CAVHD therapies require both arterial and venous circulation. Although Scribner shunts (see Fig. 4.5) have been used for CAVH, separate catheters in the femoral artery and vein are most commonly used. Prior to placing the arterial catheter, the artery should be examined and should be free from bruits. The patency of the femoral artery and the distal arteries should be confirmed by Doppler. Special arterial catheters (usual internal diameter, 3 mm) are required and the technique for catheterization is the Seldinger technique described in Section 4.2.1. After the catheter has been inserted, the patient is confined to bed to prevent trauma to the femoral artery. Because arterial catheterization is associated with serious complications (bleeding, atheroembolization, and ischemic injury to the limb distal to the catheter), the access should be monitored continuously for complications. If a major complication develops, the catheter should be removed immediately. Because the use of an arterial catheter is associated with the above, potentially serious, complications, it should be avoided if possible.

CVVH, CVVHDF, and SLEDD have become more popular because an arterial catheter is not required. These therapies are most commonly performed with a dual-lumen venous catheter that is inserted via the Seldinger technique. Internal jugular and femoral veins are the preferred choices. The right internal jugular is the optimal insertion site; however, in patients with severe pulmonary edema or raised intracranial pressure, the femoral vein is a good alternative because it does not require lowering of the patient's head for insertion. Femoral catheters should be long enough (at least 20 cm) to reach into the inferior vena cava to improve flow and reduce recirculation during therapies. Critically ill patients can have a previously placed central venous catheter prior to hemodialysis catheter placement. Catheters in both internal jugular veins should be avoided in patients with elevated intracranial pressure because these can retard venous outflow from the head and worsen cerebral edema. Subclavian lines should generally be avoided due to the increase risk of insertion-related complications and the risk of central venous stenosis and subsequent difficulty with permanent dialysis access. However, in certain patient populations, this is the only access available. Extreme care should be taken with removal of a subclavian hemodialysis catheter, because the puncture site is not very compressible. After catheter placement, the ports should be instilled with either heparin, or 4% sodium citrate in patients unable to receive heparin, to help maintain patency of the catheter. CRRT catheters are currently recommended to be changed only if clinically indicated, and not by a predetermined schedule [6].

7.3.2 Tubing

Various configurations of tubing with filters are available. Whichever CRRT system is used, the following characteristics should be present:

- The overall length of tubing should be as short as possible to minimize resistance.
- The arterial segment should have ports for the addition of anticoagulation, for sampling of blood (both before and after the anticoagulation port), and for pre-dilution replacement fluid infusion.
- The venous segment should have a port for post-dilution replacement fluid infusion and a sampling port.
- The tubing should have a mechanism for monitoring arterial and venous pressures.
- Venovenous therapies require a pump; thus, the venous segment should have provisions for air trapping and removal.
- All connections should have strong, fail-safe, Luer-Lok connectors to prevent accidental separation and blood loss. This is particularly important in venovenous therapies where a blood pump is used.

7.3.3 Filter

Many filters are available for CRRT use, and Table 7.3 lists filters available for hemodiafiltration. For CAVH and CAVHD, the filter must have low resistance and high water permeability.

7.3.4 Replacement Fluid

For hemofiltration and hemodiafiltration, a significant part of the ultrafiltered volume may be replaced by an alternative fluid, which must be similar in composition to plasma. Replacement fluids must be approved for direct infusion and must be sterile and pyrogen free.

7.3.4.1 Composition of Replacement Fluids

There are a number of options for replacement fluid composition. These include:

– Routine IV fluids (lactated Ringers)
– Designer replacement fluids made at the institution
– Purchased premade solutions (see Table 7.4)
– Ultrapure solutions generated from dialysate "online" (see Section 7.2.7)

Simply made solutions will use Ringer's lactate, which is similar in composition to normal plasma water (with lactate as a basic ion in place of bicarbonate). In patients with lactic acidosis or those who cannot metabolize lactate, this solution should not be used.

Two solutions can be used simultaneously (preferred) or alternated.

– One liter of normal saline (0.9%) to which 6–8 mEq of calcium and 3 mEq of magnesium are added.
– One liter of 5% dextrose and 0.225% saline, to which 75 mEq of sodium bicarbonate is added. Alternatively, if dextrose is not needed, this solution could be 0.225% saline (1/2 normal saline) to which one ampule of sodium bicarbonate is added (50 mEq of sodium bicarbonate).

If the serum bicarbonate concentration starts rising, fluid bicarbonate should be decreased to 50 mEq in the second bag and the other constituents adjusted accordingly. It is important that these solutions should be used either simultaneously or in strict sequence. Additions to the bags must be carried out under sterile conditions and patients monitored closely throughout the procedure.

The problems with designer fluids are that they are resource intensive for the pharmacy to produce, there is a lag time from when they are ordered until they are available for patient use, and laboratory confirmation of the composition is required. Although premade commercially available solutions address some of these

Table 7.3 Filters for hemofiltration and hemodiafiltration

Manufacturer	Model	Material	Area (m^2)	Priming volume (ml)
B Braun	Diacap			
	PS10 High	PS	1.0	58
	PS12 High	PS	1.2	68
	PS15 High	PS	1.5	90
	PS18 High	PS	1.8	110
	PS20 High	PS	2.0	121
Baxter	Tricea			
	110G	CT	1.1	65
	150G	CT	1.5	90
	190G	CT	1.9	115
	210G	CT	2.1	125
	Exeltra			
	150	CT	1.5	95
	170	CT	1.7	105
	190	CT	1.9	115
	210 Plus	CT	2.1	125
	Syntra			
	120	PES	1.2	87
	160	PES	1.6	117
Bellcosorin	BLS			
	512	PES	1.3	77
	514	PES	1.4	85
	517	PES	1.7	99
	812	PES	1.2	73
	814	PES	1.4	85
	816	PES	1.6	94
	819	PES	1.9	109
Fresenius	Optiflux F			
	160NR	PS	1.5	84
	180A	PS	1.8	105
	200A	PS	2.0	113
	200NR	PS	2.0	113
	F			
	50S	PS	1.0	63
	60S	PS	1.3	82
	70S	PS	1.6	98
	FX			
	40	PS	0.6	32
	50	PS	1.0	53
	60	PS	1.4	74
	80	PS	1.8	95
	100	PS	2.2	116
Gambro	Polyflux			
	140H	PA	1.4	75
	170H	PA	1.7	94
	210H	PA	2.1	120

(continued)

Table 7.3 (continued)

Manufacturer	Model	Material	Area (m^2)	Priming volume (ml)
	17R	PA	1.7	121
	21R	PA	2.1	152
	24R	PA	2.4	165
Hospal	Nephral ST			
	200	PAN	1.1	64
	300	PAN	1.3	81
	400	PAN	1.7	98
	500	PAN	2.2	126
Idemsa	MHP			
	120	PES	1.2	71
	140	PES	1.4	81
	160	PES	1.6	88
	180	PES	1.8	104
	200	PES	2.0	112
Nipro	Surelyzer PES			
	110DH	PES	1.1	68
	150DH	PES	1.5	93
	190DH	PES	1.9	118
	FB			
	150U	CT	1.5	90
	150UH	CT	1.5	90
Nikkiso	FLX			
	15GW	PP	1.5	91
	18GW	PP	1.8	108
	FDX			
	150GW	PP	1.5	91
	180GW	PP	1.8	108
	FDY			
	150GW	PP	1.5	91
	180GW	PP	1.8	108
Nephros	OLpur MD			
	190	PES	1.9	140
	220	PES	2.2	155
Toray	BK-P			
		PMMA	1.3	76
		PMMA	1.6	94
		PMMA	2.1	126
	BS			
		PS	1.3	81
		PS	1.6	102
		PS	1.8	116

PS polysulfone, CT cellulose triacetate, PES polyether sulfone, PA polyamide blend, PAN polyacrylonitrile, PP polyester polymer alloy, PMMA polymethylmethacrylate. Adapted from [7]

Table 7.4 Replacement fluids

Component	"Online" generation	PD fluid	LR	Accusol (2.5-l bag)	Prismasate (5-l bag)	Prismasate-L (5-l bag)	NxStage 1 (5-l bag)	NxStage 2 (5-l bag)	Normocarb
Sodium (mEq/l)	Variable	132	130	140	140	140	140	140	140
Potassium (mEq/l)	Variable	0	4	0, 2, 4	0, 2, 4	0	0, 2, 4	1, 3	0
Chloride (mEq/l)	Variable	96	109	109.5–116.3	108–120.5	109	109–113	100–112	106
Bicarbonate (mEq/l)	Variable	0	0	30, 35	22, 32	0	35	0	35
Calcium (mEq/l)	Variable	3.5	2.7	2.8, 3.5	0, 2.5, 3.5	2.5	3	3	0
Magnesium (mEq/l)	0.75	0.5	0	1, 1.5	1, 1.5	1.5	1	1	1.5
Lactate (mEq/l)	2	40	28	0	3	35	0	35, 40, 45	0
Glucose (mg/dl)	100	1,360		0, 110	0, 110	110	100	100	0

PD fluid, peritoneal dialysis fluid from Baxter Healthcare Corp., McGraw Park, IL; LR lactated Ringer's solution. Accusol, Baxter Healthcare Corp.; Prismasate, Gambro Renal Products, Lakewood, CO; NxStage, NxStage Medical Inc., Lawrence MA; Normocarb, B. Braun Medical Inc., Bethlehem, PA. Adapted from [7]

issues, they are more expensive and often flexibility is lost. "Online" generation of replacement fluids, from ultrapure dialysate, solves the complexity and expense problems. However, these systems are still undergoing clinical trials in the USA in early 2008.

7.3.4.2 Site of Replacement Fluids

As discussed above, the ultrafiltered volume can be replaced by infusion of replacement fluid into the arterial segment (prefilter, pre-dilution) or into the venous segment (postfilter, post-dilution) of the tubing set.

pre-dilution: This is useful if a large volume of ultrafiltrate has to be removed, because substantial UF without pre-dilution can cause significant hemoconcentration in the later part of filter and the adjacent tubing segment, increasing the risk of clotting. With pre-dilution, however, the urea concentrations in the plasma after the addition of replacement fluid are about 10–20% lower than in the plasma prior to the addition of fluid, thus, clearance of urea is relatively lower. The pre-dilution method should be preferred if the hematocrit is greater than 40% or if the UF rate is >10ml/min (Table 7.5). The volume of replacement fluid is equal to the UF volume minus the weight loss required; however, the UF volume required to get similar urea clearance is about 10–15% larger for pre-dilution than for post-dilution.

post-dilution: This method requires a relatively smaller volume of ultrafiltrate and replacement fluid. In post-dilution hemofiltration, the clearance of urea is equal to the ultrafiltration rate because the urea concentration in the ultrafiltrate is equal to the plasma urea concentration. The volume required is equal to the UF volume minus the weight loss required.

Table 7.5 Comparison of pre-dilution and post-dilution guidelines

Site of Replacement Fluid	Advantages	Disadvantages	Indications
pre-dilution	Reduced clotting	Requires larger volume of replacement fluid	UFR >10ml/min
	Faster UFR		Hematocrit >40% No/low anticoagulation Increased clotting
post-dilution	Less volume of replacement fluid	Limited UFR	No specific indication; can be used under all conditions other than listed above
		May increase clotting risk	
	No hemodilution Good clearance		

UFR ultrafiltration rate

The following example demonstrates the difference in clearance when comparing pre-dilution with post-dilution strategies.

Assume a patient with 45 l of total body water requires an UF volume and replacement fluid (RF) volume of 40 l/day, or 28 ml/min, and a blood flow (Qb) of 140 ml/min. What is the percent dilution with a prefilter replacement fluid infusion?

% Dilution = RF (ml/min)/[Qb (ml/min) + RF (ml/min)]
% Dilution = 28 ml/min/(140 + 28) mL/min
% Dilution = 28/168
% Dilution = 16.5%

Now assume an additional 5-l ultrafiltration for volume overload, calculate the Kt/V with pre-dilution or post-dilution replacement fluids, where K is the dialyzer urea clearance, t is the duration of dialysis, and V is the volume of distribution of urea.
RF at 40 l/day + UF at 5 l/day = 45 l/day total volume
post-dilution

Kt = 45 l
V = 45 l
Kt/V = 45/45 = 1

pre-dilution

Kt = 45 l + 16.5% dilution = 37.5 l
V = 45 l
Kt/V = 37.5/45 = 0.83

7.3.5 Dialysis Fluid

Increased porosity of the hemofilters requires that the dialysate used must be sterile and pyrogen free. Commercially available peritoneal dialysis (PD) solutions are commonly used in counter-current flow through the filter to allow diffusion of solutes. PD solutions are potassium free, and potassium may need to be added to prevent hypokalemia. The solutions are dextrose-rich and, as such, significant quantities of dextrose can diffuse into the blood. The calories from dialysate dextrose should be taken into account when calculating the caloric requirements of the patient. With the use of PD solution-based dialysate, the replacement fluid is generally kept dextrose free.

Patients with liver disease and/or severe acidosis may not be able to metabolize lactate-based PD or NxStage solutions and may require a bicarbonate-based dialysate. An increase in anion gap and no improvement in acidosis should suggest that the lactate load is not being metabolized and a change to a bicarbonate-based dialysate may be necessary. It should be noted that lower bicarbonate concentrations are generally used when regional citrate anticoagulation is used because the citrate metabolism yields bicarbonate.

Alternatively, the replacement fluids manufactured as premade solutions can also be used as dialysate (see Table 7.4), or the local pharmacy can prepare dialysate-like solutions. "Online" generation of replacement fluid from ultrapure dialysate is used in Europe but at this time does not have regulatory approval in the United States.

SLEDD uses a regular dialyzer, thus, the usual commercially available conventional A and B baths of HD can be used.

7.3.6 Machines

A number of machines are available for CRRT therapies. The five integrated hemofiltration CRRT systems available in the United States are:

- Accura®, Baxter Healthcare, Deerfield, IL
- Diapact®, B. Braun, Bethlehem, PA
- Prisma®, Gambro, Lakewood, CO
- PrismaFlex®, Gambro, Lakewood, CO
- System One®, NxStage Medical, Lawrence, MA

Of these, all but NxStage can also perform hemodiafiltration. For SLEDD, Fresenius 2008K and 2008H machines are used, quite often along with the Gambro 200S Ultra.

7.4 Dialysate Flow and Ultrafiltration Rates

Dialysate flow and UF rates depend on the desired clearance of urea or creatinine by combined diffusive and convective transports. The following example illustrates this and can be used to calculate dialysate flow and UF rate.

Example

A patient with acute renal failure is evaluated on a Monday at 07:00. The patient's usual (dry) weight is 62 kg but on Monday his weight is 70 kg and his blood urea nitrogen (BUN) is 60 mg/dl. His weight and BUN are reevaluated 24 h later, during which time he has gained 2 kg, his BUN has risen to 80 mg/dl, and he has taken 3 l of water and voided 500 ml of urine (which contained 3 g of urea). The patient is expected to get 3 l fluids in next 24 h but no additional losses are anticipated. To begin CVVHD, dialysate flow and UF rate must be calculated.

Step 1—Calculation of urea generation rate

Urea content on Monday = BUN × volume of distribution
$$= 0.60 \text{g/l} \times [(0.6 \times 621) + (0.60 \text{g/l} \times 8l)] = 27.12 \text{g}$$

(Volume of distribution of urea = 60% dry weight + extracellular volume (ECV) excess weight on Monday = 70 kg, of which, about 8 l is ECV excess and 10 l on Tuesday includes 2 l of weight gain from Monday).

Urea content on Tuesday $= 0.80 \text{g/l} \times [(0.6 \times 621) + (0.8 \text{g/l} \times 10l)] = 37.76 \text{g}$

Urea in the urine in 24 h = 3 g. Urea generated between Monday and Tuesday (24 h) = increase in urea content + urea lost in urine + urea lost in other fluid losses.

$$= (37.76 - 27.12) + 3 + 0 \text{g}$$
$$= 13.64 \text{g in 24 h}$$

Step 2—Calculation of urea clearance required to maintain urea concentration in a certain range

Suppose the goal is to maintain BUN at an 80 mg/dl level for the next 24 h (assuming the same urea generation and losses).

Urea nitrogen removal = urea nitrogen generation (to maintain status quo)
= 13.64 g/24 h (from Step 1)
Urea removal = urea clearance × urea concentration
13.64 g/24 h = urea clearance 1/24 h × 0.8 g/l
Or, urea clearance = 13.64(g/24 h)/0.8(g/l) = 17.05 l/24 h

Step 3—Calculation of UF and replacement fluid rates for CVVH or CAVH

A. post-dilution hemofiltration:

Total UF volume = UF for urea clearance (ignoring the effect of urinary and other fluid losses on urea removal) + anticipated fluid infusion = 17.05 (from Step 2) + 3 = 20.05 l/24 h.
Total replacement fluid = total UF volume + urine loss + other fluid losses (e.g., gastric suction) − desired weight loss − anticipated fluid infusion
= 20.05 + 0.5 + 0 − 2 − 3 = 15.5 l/day
Replacement fluid (post-dilution) = 15.5 l/day

B. pre-dilution hemofiltration:

UF volume to get desired urea clearance with pre-dilution = urea clearance $\times 1.15 = 17.05 \times 1.15 = 19.6L$ (15% lower urea concentration due to pre-dilution)

Replacement fluid = UF volume + urine loss + other losses (e.g., gastric suction) $= 19.6 + 0.5 + 0 = 20.1 l/day$

Total UF volume = replacement fluid + desired weight loss + anticipated fluid infusion $= 20.1 + 2 + 3 = 25.1 l/day$

C. Combined CVVHDF:

With slow dialysate flow rates of $< 150 ml/min$, the dialysate concentration of urea = plasma concentration of urea. Thus, the urea clearance (clearance = $D/P \times V$) = dialysate flow rate + UF rate $= 17.05 l/day$ (from Step 2). This can be divided between the dialysate and UF rates.

If the dialysate flow is 10 l/day, then the UF rate $= 7.05 l +$ the volume to maintain fluid balance.

Fluid to maintain fluid balance = anticipated fluid infusion + desired weight loss−urine and other losses $= 3 l + 2 l - 0.5 l = 4.5 l/day$

$UF = 7.05 + 4.5 = 11.55 l/day$

Thus, for post-dilution CVVHDF, dialysate flow rate = 10 l/day, UF rate = 11.55 l/day, and replacement fluid rate = 7.05 l/day.

Divide the total clearance volume between the UF and dialysate flows.

Replacement fluid = UF rate weight − loss desired.

This and other examples are given only to illustrate the concept. They cannot be used as a guide to therapy. Other clinical variables must be considered and treatment modified accordingly.

7.5 Anticoagulation

Anticoagulation during continuous therapies can be quite challenging. Objectives for anticoagulation include:

– 24- to 48-h system and filter patency; frequent clotting of the filter increases the cost and clotted fibers limit the efficiency of the system
– Minimum systemic anticoagulation to reduce the risk of bleeding. It is difficult and challenging to achieve the correct balance between this and filter patency
– An anticoagulant with minimum side effects and a short half-life, which can be reversed easily if necessary
– Simple and inexpensive monitoring of the level of anticoagulation

Several anticoagulation methods have been used, but an ideal method has not yet been found.

7.5.1 Heparin

Heparin is the most commonly used anticoagulant, and many different methods of heparinization have been proposed. Filters can be prerinsed with heparin, and heparin is generally infused into the arterial limb of the extracorporeal circuit in doses of 500–2,000 U as a loading dose and then maintained as a continuous infusion at 300–500 U/h (5–10 U/kg/h) rate. Hourly adjustments are made to keep the partial thrombin time (a PTT) or activated clotting time 1.25–2.0 times baseline. Bleeding complications are common with prolonged treatments.

7.5.2 Low Molecular Weight Heparin

Experience with low molecular weight heparin (LMWH; heparin fractions in the 4- to 7-kDa range) in CRRT is limited [8]. LMWH produces an anticoagulant effect predominantly through antifactor X activity. With the lower nonspecific binding, LMWH has a more favorable profile of bleeding. However, it generally has a long half-life and is cleared via the kidneys, leading to even longer half-lives in renal failure.

A metaanalysis of 11 trials of LMWH versus unfractionated heparin in IHD and hemofiltration found that bleeding events were not significantly different with LMWH [9]. Fixed-dose dalteparin has been shown to provide identical filter life, comparable safety in terms of bleeding, but increased total daily cost, including coagulation assays, compared with adjusted-dose heparin in CRRT in an adult intensive care unit (ICU) [10].

7.5.3 Citrate

Citrate binds with calcium to form a complex that is readily removed by diffusion dialysis. It is an effective procedure that provides desired regional anticoagulation. The circuits are free of clots and there is no risk of excessive bleeding. With prolonged infusion, particularly with CVVH, citrate toxicity is common, leading to hypocalcemia/hypercalcemia, hypomagnesemia, hypernatremia, and metabolic alkalosis. Citrate use is safer when diffusion dialysis is being used. To prevent hypernatremia, the dialysate sodium should be decreased and the amount of bicarbonate or lactate in the dialysate and/or replacement fluid also decreased. Four percent trisodium citrate solution containing citrate (140 mmol/l) can be infused into the

Table 7.6 Anticoagulant citrate dextrose form A (ACD-A) citrate and calcium titration guidelines

Postfilter ionized calcium (mM)	Adjustment of ACD-A rate
< 0.20	Reduce rate by 5 ml/h
0.20–0.40	No adjustment
0.40–0.50	Increase rate by 5 ml/h
> 0.50	Increase rate by 10 ml/h

Calcium chloride infusion titrated to systemic ionized calcium level

Systemic ionized calcium (mmol/l)	Adjustments of calcium infusion
> 1.45	Reduce rate by 10 ml/h
1.21–1.45	Reduce rate by 5 ml/h
1.01–1.20	No adjustment
0.90–1.00	Increase rate by 5 ml/h
< 0.90	10 mg/kg calcium chloride bolus; increase rate by 10 ml/h

Adapted from [13]

arterial line at a rate of 170 ml/h [11, 12]. Hypocalcemia can be avoided by adjusting the calcium concentration of the dialysate and/or of the replacement fluid. Table 7.6 demonstrates a citrate–calcium titration protocol:

7.5.3.1 Citrate Dialysate

Citrasate$^{®}$ dialysate (Advanced Renal Technologies, Bellevue, WA), a citric acid-based dialysate, is a new option for anticoagulation during hemodialysis. This formulation uses citric acid at 2.4 mEq/l as the primary acidifying agent in the "A" bath with 0.3 mEq/l acetate. Citrate dialysate has been shown to be well tolerated during SLEDD runs both in the general ICU population [14] and in patients with advanced liver failure [15]. It has also been successfully used for intraoperative dialysis during orthotopic liver transplantation [16].

7.5.4 Prostacyclin

Prostacyclin (PGI_2) inhibits platelet aggregation and is a potent anticoagulant. However, it causes hypotension, is expensive, requires monitoring by platelet aggregation studies, and has a prolonged antiplatelet effect (without the means to reverse it). It has been used with good results in a small number of pediatric patients [17]. Epoprostenol has also been used as the sole anticoagulant in CVVH patients (n = 51), with 1.0 bleeding episode per 1,000 patient-hours of treatment. The median life span of the extracorporeal circuit was 15 h [18]. Another study demonstrated that regional citrate anticoagulation offered longer filter survival as compared with combined prostacyclin and heparin in CVVH. The regional citrate was also cheaper [19]. Prostacyclin may offer longer filter survival and be associated with less bleeding risk than unfractionated heparin during CRRT in high-risk bleeding patients [20, 21]. Prostacyclin should be avoided in patients with fulminant hepatic failure because its infusion may increase intracerebral pressure and thus decrease cerebral perfusion pressure in this group of patients at risk of dying from cerebral edema [22, 23]. Critically ill patients with respiratory failure can develop worsening ventilatory/perfusion mismatches with subsequent decreased oxygen delivery and uptake [24]. With the above concerns, prostacyclin should be used with extreme care for CRRT.

7.5.5 Argatroban

Argatroban is a direct thrombin inhibitor that is metabolized by the liver but not cleared by the kidneys. There is little data on the safety and efficacy of argatroban in CRRT. One of the largest reported studies looked at 47 patients, including 14 patients on CRRT, and found bleeding events in 6% of the treatments (n = 50) [25]. A recommended dosing guideline is given in Table 7.7. Of note, argatroban will artificially raise the International Normalized Ratio for prothrombin activity (INR), and thus activated partial thromboplastin time (aPTT) is followed. Overdoses are treated with administration of fresh frozen plasma.

7.5.6 Lepirudin

Lepirudin, a recombinant hirudin, is also a direct thrombin inhibitor that is renally cleared. See Table 7.7 for dosing. Of note, antibodies to lepirudin may develop after 5 days of use, leading to a potentiation of its anticoagulant effect. There is no effective antidote; however, there is a case report of activated factor VIIa being used for hirudin-induced postoperative bleeding [26]. Data is also limited to its use in CRRT.

7.5.7 Danaparoid

Danaparoid, a heparinoid of low molecular weight (5.5 kDa) consisting of heparan sulfate (83%), dermatan sulfate, and chondroitin sulfate, has been used for CRRT anticoagulation but is currently unavailable for use in the United States.

Table 7.7 Anticoagulation alternatives

	Priming dose	Maintenance dose	Notes
Heparin	500–2,000 U	250–500 U/h	Maintain arterial aPTT > 45 s and venous > 60 s; increase or decrease by 100 U/h as needed
LMWH	40 mg	10–40 mg/h	Prolonged half life, different LMWHs may need differing doses
Regional citrate	See Table 7.6		
Citrate dialysate	Connect the acid concentrate to the machine		
Prostacyclin		4–8 mg/kg/min	Watch in cerebral edema and severe V/Q mismatches
Argatroban		0.5–1.0 μg/kg/min	Start lower with liver dysfunction. Follow aPTT, $1.25 - 2.0\times$ baseline
Lepirudin		0.005–0.001 mg/kg/h	Follow aPTT, $1.5 - 2.0\times$ baseline
Nafamostat		0.1 mg/kg/h	Little experience
Saline flushes		100 ml flush each 30 min	Can use in conjunction with low-dose heparin in patients with elevated bleeding risk

aPTT activated partial thromboplastin time, *LMWH* low molecular weight heparin

7.5.8 Fondaparinux

Fondaparinux is a synthetic pentasaccharide that inhibits factor Xa by binding to antithrombin. Although it has been used in IHD [27], its use in CRRT needs further evaluation. Its anticoagulant properties are monitored by measuring antifactor Xa activity. A major drawback is its half-life, which is longer than the LMWH and lengthens further in renal failure.

7.5.9 Nafamostat

Nafamostat, a synthetic serine protease inhibitor used mainly in Japan, has an extremely short half-life (5–8 min). A dose of 0.1 mg/kg/h in CAVH and CAVHD is reported to prevent clotting and carries a very low risk of bleeding [28]. It should not be used with negatively charged membranes because the drug can be absorbed by the membrane [29].

7.5.10 No Anticoagulation

In patients with prolonged bleeding times, thrombocytopenia, and liver failure, increased bleeding risk has led to the use of continuous therapies without anticoagulation. Despite prolonged bleeding times in these patients, the system usually clots and the filter needs to be changed after about 8 h. When using CRRT without anticoagulation, using a pre-dilution technique, increasing the dialysate flow to 3 l/h, and periodic saline flushes can help decrease clotting.

7.6 Drug Removal During CRRT

Data regarding the clearance of drugs during continuous therapies continues to grow. The following factors are known to influence drug removal:

Therapy-related factors

– UF rate
– Dialysate flow rate

Drug-related factors

– Molecular weight of the drug
– Protein binding
– Volume of distribution
– Endogenous clearance

For continuous hemofiltration alone, the UF rate can be considered to be equivalent to the glomerular filtration rate (GFR); the dose adjustment information for that degree of GFR can be used. For example, if a patient is undergoing 600 ml/h UF (10 ml/min) without any dialysis, then the loss of a drug would be similar to that seen in patients with a GFR of 10 ml/min. The addition of dialysis makes this estimation more difficult because the diffusive clearances of drugs are different. Table 7.8 shows the sieving coefficients of some commonly used drugs. The clearance of a drug is equal to the UF rate multiplied by the sieving coefficient. If possible, the drug level should be monitored and the dose adjusted accordingly. In addition to

Table 7.8 Sieving coefficients of some common drugs

Drug	Sieving coefficient (UF/P)	Drug	Sieving coefficient (UF/P)
Amikacin	0.88	Imipenum	0.80
Amphotericin	0.40	Metronidazole	0.86
Ampicillin	0.69	Moxalactam	0.44
Cefoperazone	0.27	Nafcillin	0.54
Cefotaxime	0.51	Oxacillin	0.02
Cefoxitin	0.64	Phenytoin	0.45
Ceftazidime	0.70	Procainamide	0.86
Ceftizoxime	0.63	Streptomycin	0.30
Ceftriaxone	0.71	Procainamide (N-acetyl)	0.92
Cefuroxime	0.86	Ranitidine	0.74
Cephapirin	1.48	Theophylline	0.85
Clindamycin	0.98	Thiocyanate	1.07
Digoxin	0.96	Tobramycin	0.78
Erythromycin	0.37	Valproic acid	0.18
Gentamicin	0.81	Vancomycin	0.76

drugs, significant quantities of nutrients (as high as 15 g/day of amino acids) are also removed during continuous therapy. The net protein loss has been measured at 77 mg/dl of filtrate [4].

7.7 Intraoperative Dialysis

A number of critically ill dialysis dependent patients need to undergo emergent, often life saving, surgical procedures. In certain of these cases, the patient would not survive the surgical procedure without dialytic assistance during the surgery. These include patients undergoing liver transplantation or cardiac surgery with volume excess, significant acidemia, and/or significant electrolyte abnormalities such as hyperkalemia.

Patients undergoing liver transplantation who often require intraoperative dialysis include those who are already dialysis dependant (fulminant liver failure, hepatorenal syndrome, acute tubular necrosis, etc.) and those with impending dialysis who would not survive the underlying imbalance without dialytic support during the surgery. As stated above, indications for intraoperative dialysis include:

– Hyperkalemia
– Volume overload with associated oligoanuria
– Severe metabolic acidosis

Most patients have a temporary catheter, generally located on the right side of the neck or in the groin, requiring extended tubing to connect the catheter and machine.

The tubing runs from the access catheter under the surgical drape to the machine, generally located at the head of the bed on the right. Extra tubing sets and varying potassium baths should be available in the room as well. Although CVVHDF has been used, SLEDD therapy works extremely well and bypasses any logistic issues obtaining and changing replacement fluids during the surgery. This also allows citrate dialysate (see Section 7.5.3) to be used for extracorporeal circuit anticoagulation. Citrate dialysate is well tolerated even during the anhepatic and reperfusion states without any signs of citrate toxicity [16].

Advantages of intraoperative dialysis include:

– Volume control
– Maintenance of electrolyte homeostasis
– Stability of acid/base status
– Reversal of uremic bleeding diathesis
– Temperature control of the patient

Intraoperative dialysis with either CVVH or CVVHDF has also been used in cardiac surgery while the patient is on cardiopulmonary bypass [30, 31]. Dialytic support can also be offered to patients receiving extracorporeal membrane oxygenation (ECMO). In this case, the ECMO blood lines are connected in parallel to the dialyzer.

Intraoperative dialysis can be a life-saving procedure allowing critically ill patients to survive surgery. Differing modalities have been successfully used, with CVVH and CVVHDF in cardiac surgery cases and SLEDD therapies during orthotopic liver transplantation.

7.8 Dose of Dialysis in Continuous Therapies

The ideal dose of dialysis for CRRT is unknown. However, a number of randomized control studies have been undertaken to begin the process of elucidating the ideal dose of dialysis in the ICU population. Ronco et al. looked at 425 patients with acute kidney injury and randomized patients to CVVH with varying ultrafiltration rates (20, 35, or 45 ml/kg/h). Fifteen-day survival was significantly lower in the 20 ml/kg/h group as compared with the other two study groups [32]. In a nonblinded, single-center study, CVVH at an UF rate of 25 ± 5 ml/kg/h was compared with CVVHDF at a UF rate of 24 ± 6 ml/kg/h and a dialysate flow of 18 ± 5 ml/kg/h. Significantly higher survival was found at 28 and 90 days with the additional solute clearance of the CVVHDF [33].

Studies are ongoing to help further delineate the answer to this question. The United States Veterans Administration (VA)/the National Institutes of Health (NIH) "Acute Renal Failure Trial Network" (ATN) study is looking at two different dialysis dose ranges for all patients requiring IHD or CRRT for acute tubular necrosis. The "Intensive therapy" arm undergoes IHD or SLEDD therapy six times per week with a target Kt/V of 1.2 to 1.4 per treatment. If the patient requires continuous therapy, the UF rate target is 35 ml/kg/h. The "Less intensive therapy" arm undergoes IHD or SLEDD therapies three times per week or a UF rate of 20 ml/kg/h for continuous therapies [34]. The second ongoing study, in Australia and New Zealand, looking at 25 vs 40 ml/kg/h UF rates in CVVHDF [35].

Additionally, a pair of meta-analyses have recently been published addressing this question [36, 37].

While awaiting further definitive studies focusing on the desired dose of dialysis needed in the ICU, we recommend aiming for IHD Kt/V of 1.2 per session and CVVH ultrafiltration rates of 35 ml/kg/h to ensure that these critically ill patients receive adequate dialysis.

References

1. Kramer P, Wigger W, Reiger J, et al. Arteriovenous hemofiltration: a new and simple method for treatment of over-hydrated patients resistant to diuretics. *Klin Wochenschr.* 1977; 55:1121–1122.
2. Tominaga GT, Ingegno M, Cerldi C, Waxman K. Vascular complications of continuous arteriovenous hemofiltration in trauma patients. *J Trauma.*1993; 35:285.
3. Bellomo R, Parkin G, Love J, Boyce, N. A prospective comparative study of continuous arteriovenous hemodiafiltration and continuous venovenous hemodiafiltration in critically ill patients. *Am J Kidney Dis.* 1993; 21:400.
4. Kaplan AA. Continuous arteriovenous hemofiltration and related therapies. In: *Replacement of Renal Function by Dialysis.* 4th edition. Edited by C Jacobs, CM Kjellstrand, KM Koch and JF Winchester. Dordrecht: Kluwer, 1993, pp. 390–418.
5. Tam, PY-W, Huraib S, Mahan B, et al. Slow continuous hemodialysis for the management of acute renal failure in an intensive care unit. *Clin Nephrol.* 1988; 30:79.
6. *CDC Guidelines for the Prevention of Intravascular Catheter-Related Infections.* MMWR August 9, 2002/51(RR10), pp. 1–26.
7. Daugirdas JT, Blake PG, Ing TS. *Handbook of Dialysis,* 4th edition. Philadelphia, PA: Lippincott William & Wilkins, 2007.
8. Shrader J, Scheler F. Coagulation disorders in acute renal failure and anticoagulation during CAVH with standard heparin and LMW heparin. In: *Continuous Arteriovenous Hemofiltration.* Edited by HG Sieberth and H Mann. Basel: Karger, 1985, pp. 25–55.
9. Lim W, Cook DJ, Crowther MA. Safety and efficacy of low molecular weight heparins for hemodialysis in patients with end-stage renal failure: A meta-analysis of randomized trials. *J Am Soc Nephrol.* 2004; 15:3192–3206.
10. Reeves JH, Cumming AR, Gallagher L, et al. A controlled trial of low-molecular-weight heparin (dalteparin) versus unfractionated heparin as anticoagulant during continuous venovenous hemodialysis with filtrations. *Crit Care Med.* 1999; 27:2224–2228.
11. Ahmad S, Yeo KT, Jensen WM, et al. Citrate anticoagulation during in vivo simulation of slow hemofiltration. *Blood Purif.* 1990; 8:177–182.
12. Mehta RL, McDonald BR, Aguilar MM, et al. Regional citrate anticoagulation for continuous arteriovenous hemodialysis in critically ill patients. *Kidney Int.* 1990; 38:976–981.
13. Swartz R, et al. Improving the delivery of continuous renal replacement therapy using regional citrate anticoagulation. *Clin Nephrol.* 2004; 61:134–143.
14. Tu A, et al. Heparin Free Slow Low Efficiency Dialysis (SLED) Using Citrate Dialysate Is Safe and Effective. Poster presented at the 12th International Conference on Continuous Renal Replacement Therapies (CRRT) March 7–10, 2007, San Diego, CA.
15. Tu A, et al. Citrate Dialysate in SLED Is Safe and Effective in the Presence of Severe Liver Dysfunction. Poster presented at the European Renal Association and European Dialysis and Transplant Association Congress, Barcelona, Spain, June 2007.

16. Winrow RM, Tu A, Ahmad S. Intra-operative dialysis during liver transplantation for fulminant liver failure using citrate dialysate. European Renal Association-European Dialysis and Transplant Association Annual Congress. Stockholm, Sweden. May 10–13, 2008.

17. Zobel G, Trop M, Muntean W, et al. Anticoagulation for continuous arteriovenous hemofiltration in children. *Blood Purif.* 1988; 6:90–95.

18. Fiaccadori E, Maggiore U, Rotelli C, Minari M, Melfa L, Cappe G, Cabassi A. Continuous hemofiltration in acute renal failure with prostacyclin as the sole anti-hemostatic agent. *Intensive Care Med.* 2002; 28:586–593.

19. Balik M, Waldauf P, Plasil P, Pachl J. Prostacyclin versus citrate in continuous hemofiltration: an observational study in patients with high risk of bleeding. *Blood Purif.* 2005; 232:325–329.

20. Davenport A, Will EJ, Davison AM. Comparison of the use of standard heparin and prostacyclin anticoagulation in spontaneous and pump-driven extracorporeal circuits in patients with combined acute renal and hepatic failure. *Nephron.* 1994; 66:431–437.

21. Kozek-Langenecke SA, Spiss CK, Gamsjager T, Domenig C, Zimpfer M. Anticoagulation with prostaglandins and unfractionated heparin during continuous venovenous hemofiltrations: a randomized controlled trial. *Wien Klin Wochenschr.* 2002; 114:96–101.

22. Davenport A, Will EJ, Davison AM. The effect of prostacyclin on intracranial pressure in patients with acute hepatic and renal failure. *Clin Nephrol.* 1991; 35:151–157.

23. Davenport A, Will EJ, Davison AM. Adverse effects on cerebral perfusion of prostacyclin administration directly into patients with fulminant hepatic failure and acute renal failure. *Nephron.* 1991; 59:449–454.

24. Davenport A, Will EJ, Davison AM. Adverse effects of prostacyclin administered directly into patients with combined renal and respiratory failure prior to dialysis. *Intensive Care Med.* 1990; 16:431–435.

25. Reddy BV, Grossman EJ, Trevino SA, Hursting MJ, Murray PT. Argatroban anticoagulation in patients with heparin-induced thrombocytopenia requiring renal replacement therapy. *Ann Pharmacother.* 2005; 39:1601–1605.

26. Hein OV, Heymann C, Morgera S, Konertz W, Ziemer S, Spies C. Protracted bleeding after hirudin anticoagulation for cardiac surgery in a patient with HIT II and chronic renal failure. *Artif Organs.* 2005; 29:507–510.

27. Flanigan MJ, Von Brecht J, Freeman RM, Lin VS. Reducing the hemorrhagic complications of hemodialysis: A controlled comparison of low-dose heparin and citrate anticoagulation. *Am J Kidney Dis.* 1987; 9:147–153.

28. Ohtake Y, Hirasawa H, Sugai T, et al. A study on anticoagulants in continuous hemofiltration. *Jpn J Artif Organs.* 1990; 19:744.

29. Inagaki O, Nishian Y, Iwaki R, Nakagawa K, Takamitsu Y, Fujita Y. Adsorption of nafamostat mesylate by hemodialysis membranes. *Artif Organs.* 1992; 16:553–558.

30. Miyahara K, Maeda M, Sakurai H, Nakayama M, Murayama H, Hasegawa H. Cardiovascular surgery in patients on chronic dialysis: effect of intraoperative hemodialysis. *Inter Cardiovas Thorac Surg* 2004; 3:148–152.

31. Fukumoto A, Yamagishi M, Kiyoshi D, Ogawa M, Inoue T, Hashimoto S, Yaku H. Hemodiafiltration during cardiac surgery in patients on chronic hemodialysis. *J Card Surg.* 2006; 21:553–558.

32. Ronco C, Bellomo R, Homel P, Brendolan A, Dan M, Piccinni P, La Greca G. Effects of different doses in continuous veno-venous hemofiltration on outcomes of acute renal failure: a prospective randomized trail. *Lancet.* 2000; 356(9223):26–30.

33. Saudan P, Niederberger M, De Seigneux S, Ramand J, Pugin J, Perneger T, Martin PY. Adding a dialysis dose to continuous hemofiltration increases survival in patients with acute renal failure. *Kidney Int.* 2006; 70(7):1312–7.

34. Palevsky PM, O'Connor T, Zhang JH, Star RA, Smith MW. Design of the VA/NIH Acute Renal Failure Trial Network (ATN) Study: intensive versus conventional renal support in acute renal failure. *Clin Trials.* 2005; 2(5):423–35.

35. Bellomo R. Do we know the optimal dose for renal replacement therapy in the intensive care unit? *Kidney Int.* 2006; 70(7):1202–1204.

36. Bagshaw SM, Berthiaume LR, Delaney A, Bellomo R. Continuous versus intermittent renal replacement therapy for critically ill patients with acute kidney injury: A meta-analysis. *Crit Care Med.* 2008; 36(2):610–617.
37. Pannu N, Klarenbach S, Wiebe N, Manns B, Tonelli M. for the Alberta Kidney Disease Network. Renal replacement therapy in patients with acute renal failure: A systematic review. *JAMA.* 2008; 299(7):793–805.

Chapter 8
Peritoneal Dialysis

8.1 Historical Background

The first article on the use of the peritoneal cavity in experimental uremia (induced in guinea pigs) was published in 1923 by Ganter [1]. In 1961, Boen described the use of intermittent peritoneal dialysis (IPD) in patients with chronic renal failure [2]; dialysis fluid was infused into the peritoneal cavity and drained out intermittently. During the waiting period between infusion and drainage (dwell time), the solute molecules moved between the peritoneal capillaries and peritoneal fluid. This technique was effective, but cumbersome and uncomfortable because the catheter was inserted before and removed after each procedure, requiring repeated puncture of the abdominal wall. Tenckhoff [3] later developed an indwelling catheter, which led to nightly dialysis. This intermittent method, using a cycler to infuse and drain fluid while the patient slept, was the most common form of peritoneal dialysis (PD) from the 1960s to the late 1970s. In 1976, Popovich et al. [4] introduced continuous ambulatory PD (CAPD), where four to six exchanges are done each day with long dwell times between exchanges. In 1978, this group described their early clinical experience using bottled dialysis fluid. In the same year, Oreopoulos et al. [5] also described their experience with CAPD. From this point on, use of CAPD increased and cycler–IPD declined. In 1979, the Seattle group used a combination of cyclic and automated PD in two patients. This technique was called continuous automated ambulatory PD (CAAPD) [6]. In 1981, Diaz-Buxo and coworkers [7] described their more extensive experience and called this technique continuous cycling PD (CCPD)—a name that is still widely used.

8.2 Anatomy and Physiology

A basic understanding of the anatomy and physiology of the peritoneal cavity is helpful in the management of patients using the technique of PD. This understanding also helps in improving the dialysis kinetics. The peritoneal cavity is a potential

S. Ahmad, *Manual of Clinical Dialysis*, DOI 10.1007/978-0-387-09651-3_8,
© Springer Science+Business Media LLC 2009

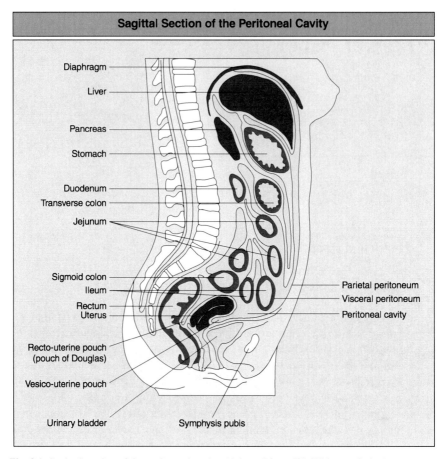

Fig. 8.1 Sagittal section of the peritoneal cavity. (Adapted from [8]. With permission)

space lined by the peritoneal membrane (see Fig. 8.1) [8], the total surface area of which approximates the surface area of the skin in adults (children have a proportionately larger surface area). The surface of the membrane is lined by a layer of lubricated mesothelial cells, beneath which lies the interstitium (containing connective tissue and blood vessels, see Fig. 8.2) [9]. The blood supply to the visceral peritoneum is derived from celiac, superior, and inferior mesenteric arteries and their local branches, while neighboring arteries supply the parietal peritoneum. The exact blood flow to the membrane is unknown but is probably from 60–70 ml/min (no greater than 200 ml/min). Venous blood drains ultimately into the hepatic portal vein. Lymphatic drainage from the peritoneal cavity is largely through the diaphragm to the lymphatics that are associated with the internal mammary and anterior mediastinal lymph nodes; ultimately draining into the right lymphatic duct. In addition, the lymphatic system from the peritoneal cavity (particularly from the omentum) also drains into the thoracic duct. The peritoneal membrane has several size pores for the movement of various molecules. There are numerous ultrasmall

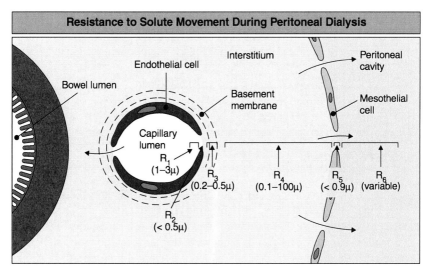

Fig. 8.2 $R1$–$R6$ represent hypothetical sites of resistance to solute movement: $R1$–$R3$, related to capillaries—blood flow, endothelium, and basement membrane; $R4$ and $R5$, peritoneal membrane—interstitium and mesothelium; and R6, peritoneal dialysate flow (reproduced from [9] with permission)

pores (0.8 nm in radius) that are transcellular (aquaporin), these mostly transport water molecules; there are many intercellular small pores (4–6 nm), which mostly transport small solutes; and there are few large pores (>20 nm) transporting only large molecules such as peptides and proteins.

8.3 Kinetics of Peritoneal Transport

Figure 8.2 shows the path of molecules between blood in the capillaries of the peritoneal membrane and dialysate fluid in the peritoneal cavity, and the various resistances to this movement. The mechanisms involved in this movement of molecules are discussed below.

8.3.1 Diffusion

As discussed in Chapter 1, the movement of solute molecules from higher concentration to side with lower concentration is called diffusion. Thus, molecules such as urea, creatinine, vitamin B_{12}, and PO_4 diffuse from blood to dialysate—where the initial concentration of these substances is zero. Glucose and lactate are present in higher concentration in the dialysate and thus diffuse into the blood. The factors affecting the diffusion are:

Concentration gradient between dialysate and blood; the larger the gradient the faster the diffusion

Effective surface area and permeability of the membrane; the higher the value the faster the diffusion

Sum of all the resistances to the path of the diffusing molecule; the larger the value the slower the diffusion

8.3.2 Ultrafiltration

Movement of solvent (water) molecules across the peritoneal membrane controlled by the pressure gradient is called ultrafiltration (UF). The hydraulic pressure gradient between the dialysate and the blood (and perhaps the lymphatics) is the major determinant of UF, but other factors, such as membrane surface area and hydraulic permeability, also are important. The hydraulic pressure in the capillary is exerted by the capillary hydrostatic pressure and is balanced by the oncotic pressure. The UF force in the peritoneal cavity is generated by the osmotic pressure of the fluid. High concentrations of dextrose in the dialysate cause a higher osmotic pressure in the cavity, drawing water out of the capillaries. The fluid flux can be expressed by the following equation:

$$J_F = K_f([P_c + s_f] - [p_c + P_f]),$$

where J_F = net solvent movement between capillaries and peritoneal fluid; K_f = peritoneal membrane permeability coefficient (surface area × permeability); P_c = hydraulic pressure in the capillary; s_f = osmotic pressure of the peritoneal fluid (dialysate); p_c = oncotic pressure in the capillary; and P_f = hydraulic pressure of the fluid in the peritoneal cavity.

8.3.2.1 Convective Solute Transport

As discussed in Chapter 1, with UF of solvent (water), solute molecules move in bulk (solvent drag). This process is called convection. The convective movement contributes significantly to the solute movement for the PD technique, particularly for the larger molecular weight substances (such as the middle molecule [MM]).

8.3.2.2 Net Ultrafiltration

Net UF is the difference in the volume of fluid infused into the peritoneal cavity and that drained out. This represents the sum of fluid movement out of the capillaries and lymphatics, minus the water reabsorbed into them.

$$\text{Net UF} = F_{oc} - (F_{ic} + F_{il})$$

where F_{oc} = fluid out of the capillaries into the peritoneal cavity; F_{ic} = fluid into the capillaries; and F_{il} = fluid into the lymphatics, both from the peritoneal cavity. Thus, increase in F_{oc} or decrease in F_{ic} and/or in F_{il} will increase net UF.

8.3.2.3 Lymphatic Absorption

The UF of water into the peritoneal cavity and the reabsorption into the blood and lymphatics of water is a continuous, dynamic process. The ratio of absorption in capillaries and in lymphatics is, however, a matter of controversy; some think that the lymphatic absorption is so significant that it may reduce the net daily UF by 80% [10], but others suggest that capillary absorption is predominant and that lymphatic absorption is a smaller fraction [11]. Whichever is the case, the lymphatic absorption of macromolecules is significant and may play an important role in the ratio of capillaric to lymphatic peritoneal fluid absorption.

References

1. Ganter G. Uber die Beseitigung giftiger Stoffe aus dem Blute durch Dialyse. *Muench Med Wochenschr* 1923, 70:1478–1485.
2. Boen ST. Kinetics of peritoneal dialysis. *Medicine* 1961, 40:243.
3. Tenckhoff H, Schechter H. A bacteriologically safe peritoneal access device. *Trans Am Soc Artif Intern Organs* 1968, 14:181–187.
4. Popovich RP, Moncrief JW, Decherd JF et al. The definition of a novel portable-wearable equilibrium peritoneal technique [Abstract]. *Am Soc Artif Intern Org* 1976, 22:64.
5. Oreopoulos DG, Robson M, Izatt S, et al. A simple and safe technique for continuous ambulatory peritoneal dialysis (CAPD). *Trans Am Soc Artif Intern Organs* 1978, 24:484–489.
6. Scribner BH. A current perspective on the role of intermittent versus continuous ambulatory peritoneal disease in the treatment of chronic renal failure. In *Pro Northeastern Meeting, Renal Physicians Association Symposium on Peritoneal Dialysis* 1979; 3:76–81.
7. Diaz-Buxo JA, Farmer CD, Walker PJ et al. Continuous cyclic peritoneal dialysis – A preliminary report. *Artif Organs* 1981, 5:157–161.
8. Twardowski ZJ. Physiology of Peritoneal Dialysis. In *Clinical Dialysis*, 3rd edition. edited by AR Nissensson, RN Fine, and DE Gentile. Norwalk: Appleton and Lange, 1995:322–342.
9. Nolph KD, Miller F, Rubin J et al. New directions in peritoneal dialysis concepts and applications. *Kidney Int* 1980, 18(Suppl 10):111–116.
10. Mactier RA, Khanna R, Twardowski ZJ et al. Contribution of lymphatic absorption to loss of ultrafiltration and solute clearance in continuous ambulatory peritoneal dialysis. *J Clin Invest* 1987, 80:1311–1316.
11. Rippe B, Zakaria ER. Lymphatic versus nonlymphatic fluid absorption from the peritoneal cavity as related to the peritoneal ultrafiltration capacity and sieving properties. *Blood Purif* 1992, 10:189–202.

Chapter 9
Technique of Peritoneal Dialysis

The essential elements of peritoneal dialysis (PD) are:

- A viable peritoneal cavity lined by a functional membrane (characteristics of a functional membrane are discussed in Chapter 8)
- Access to the peritoneal cavity, usually by means of an indwelling catheter
- Dialysis fluid and delivery mechanism

9.1 Peritoneal Dialysis Catheters

9.1.1 Description

Long-term PD was made a reality by the development (by Tenckhoff) of the first long-term indwelling catheter, created by adding Dacron® cuffs to the earlier silicone–rubber catheters. Modern catheters still use Tenckhoff's design or variations on it (see Table 9.1 and Fig. 9.1). The material of the catheter is either silicone rubber or polyurethane on which with Dacron cuffs are placed.

Each PD catheter is comprised of three parts:

- An intra-abdominal segment.
- A subcutaneous tunnel segment.
- An external segment.

The intra-abdominal segment has multiple small holes and an open terminal end. The subcutaneous segment has two cuffs, the outer cuff is placed just under the skin at the exit site, and the deep cuff is placed just external to the fascia covering the parietal peritoneum. The segment between the two cuffs lies in a tunnel, classically curved in shape, and running from the skin exit site to the deeper cuff (see Fig. 9.1).

S. Ahmad, *Manual of Clinical Dialysis*, DOI 10.1007/978-0-387-09651-3_9,
© Springer Science+Business Media LLC 2009

Table 9.1 Commonly used peritoneal catheters

Straight Tenckhoff	Easy to place by percutaneous technique
	Easy to remove and replace
	Rectal discomfort is more common and outflow problems are more common
Curled Tenckhoff	Same as above, but better patency and better outflow
	Does not impinge on the rectum
Swan neck	Same as straight Tenckhoff
	Tunnel must be curved
Missouri	Combination of Toronto Western and swan-neck catheter
	Can only be place and manipulated surgically
Lifecath	Can only be placed and manipulated surgically

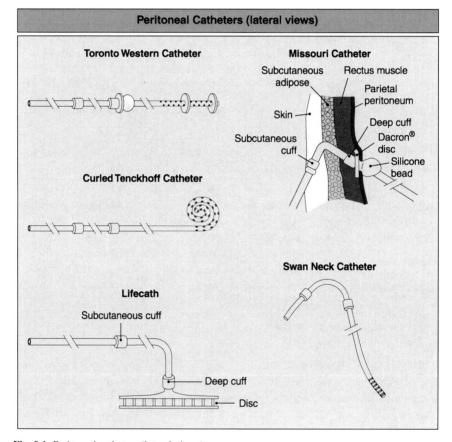

Fig. 9.1 Peritoneal catheters (lateral views)

Table 9.2 Comparison of catheter insertion techniques

Technique	Advantages	Disadvantages
Surgical	Under direct vision: Lower risk of injury to viscera Catheter placed in desired place Adhesions or large omentum can be removed surgically Any type of catheter can be inserted	More preparation is required More expensive Large incision Longer healing time
Percutaneous	Simple, easy, and quick procedure Heals quickly and can be used immediately Performed in patient's room by the nephrologist Less expensive than the other two methods	Increased risk of fluid leak Cannot be used if adhesions or large omentum present Higher failure potential
Peritoneoscopic	Faster healing Lower risk of fluid leak Simple procedure Useful even in presence of adhesions	Higher risk of injury to viscera Not all catheters can be placed by this technique Expense of the scope Training with scope.

9.1.2 Catheter Insertion Technique

Three insertion techniques are used, surgical, blind (bed side) percutaneous, and peritoneoscope (see Table 9.2). The larger catheters (Toronto Western, Lifecath, and Missouri) have to be placed surgically, but Tenckhoff catheters (straight, curved, and with or without swan neck) can be placed by any of the three techniques. Prior to insertion of the catheter, the patient should be informed of the potential complications, and the bladder and rectum should be emptied. If the patient cannot empty their bladder, a urinary catheter may be used to achieve this. This is to avoid puncturing a full bladder, particularly a potential risk during the bedside insertion.

9.1.2.1 Surgical Implantation Technique

A horizontal incision of the skin is made over the lateral border of the rectus sheath (lateral approach) or at the medial border of the rectus muscle (paramedian approach), and the subcutaneous tissue and rectus are dissected to expose the peritoneal membrane. A 1- to 2-cm-long incision is made in the parietal peritoneum, and the bowel loops, omentum, and peritoneal cavity are identified. The appropriate catheter is soaked in sterile saline (the cuffs are soaked completely), all the air

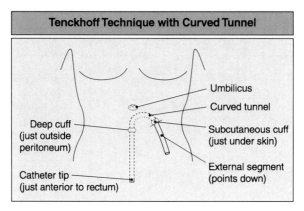

Fig. 9.2 Tenckhoff technique with curved tunnel

is squeezed out to promote growth of the tissue, and the inside of the catheter is rinsed with 30–50 ml of saline to remove particulate matter. The catheter is then placed into the peritoneal cavity, either between the anterior abdominal wall and the omentum, beneath the left inguinal ligament, or alternatively, with the tip of catheter in the pelvic space just anterior to the rectum (Tenckhoff technique, see Fig. 9.2). The peritoneum is closed around the catheter, using nonabsorbable purse-string sutures. The extent of postoperative leakage depends largely on the skill with which the peritoneum is closed. The deep cuff sits just external to the entry point through the peritoneum. Interrupted sutures are used to close the muscle and subcutaneous tissue around the deep cuff. The catheter is then laid over the skin in a curved fashion so that the external segment points down toward the feet at exit. Selection of the exit site and the length of tunnel must be performed carefully so that the external cuff lies just below it. Too much space between the cuff and the exit site increases the risk of infection, and a tunnel that is too short, over time, forces the cuff through the exit site. A tunneling tool is inserted through the exit site and advanced to the main incision, carefully tracking it to fit the shape of the desired tunnel.

The catheter is attached to the tunneling device and pulled out through the exit site until the cuff sits snugly under the site. The main incision is then closed with appropriate sutures.

9.1.2.2 Percutaneous Approach

Both straight and curved Tenckhoff's catheters can be introduced by this modification of the Tenckhoff technique. If the appropriate facilities are available, the procedure can be carried out in the patients' room (with full sterile precautions). After the patient has voided urine, the appropriate site for the primary incision is selected; either in the midline just below the umbilicus, or on the lateral side, avoiding the course of inferior and superior epigastric vessels (see Fig. 9.3). After preparing the skin and administration of local anesthesia, a 2- to 4-cm-long incision is made

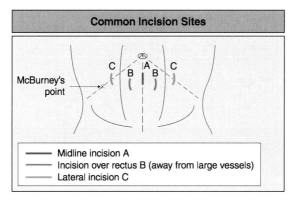

Fig. 9.3 Common incision sites

and the subcutaneous tissue is dissected down to the fascia that covers the parietal peritoneum. The patient is instructed to take a deep breath, hold it, and tense the anterior abdominal wall. A rigid Baxter Trocath (Baxter, Deerfield, IL, USA) is inserted through the peritoneum and fascia into the peritoneal cavity and the stylet is withdrawn. When this has been accomplished, the patient is allowed to breathe normally. Once the presence of the catheter in the peritoneal cavity is ensured, the cavity is filled with about 2 L of dialysate (note that in place of a Baxter catheter, a long [size 14] needle can be used to fill the peritoneal cavity). Once the cavity is full, a guide wire is fed through the catheter/needle and the catheter is then withdrawn, leaving the guide wire through the entry point into the peritoneal cavity and thus saving the entry point. The patient is again asked to tense their abdominal muscles, and a dilator with a scored, peel-away sheath is introduced over the guide wire and the insertion hole is dilated. The dilator is then removed, leaving the sheath in the cavity. A Tenckhoff catheter is threaded over the stylet, leaving about 1 cm of the internal end empty. A hemostat is applied over the stylet, just above the external end of the catheter, to prevent accidental advance of the stylet beyond the internal end of the catheter. The catheter is then advanced through the sheath (directed posteriorly), and slowly and gently angled about 20° caudally. As the tip passes through the pelvic rim, resistance to the advancement of the catheter decreases. The stylet is removed and the catheter is checked for free flow of dialysate. If the flow is not free, the catheter must be repositioned. Once the catheter is positioned in the desired place (recto-cecal pouch), the sheath is peeled away. A curved tunnel is created (as described for the surgical procedure above) and the main incision closed.

9.1.2.3 Insertion with Peritoneoscopy

This procedure (the equipment for which is available from Medigroup, Aurora, IL, USA) is especially useful if adhesions are suspected. A trocar inside a metal cannula is advanced into the peritoneal cavity of an empty abdomen. A plastic Quill guide is coiled around the cannula, the trocar is removed, and the peritoneoscope is inserted through the Quill guide; the position is confirmed by noting the smooth surface of the bowel and blood vessels, moving with respiration. The scope is removed and the abdomen is filled with 600 ml of filtered air. The scope is then reinserted through the Quill guide and the whole unit is advanced under direct vision to the most suitable place, avoiding adhesions and small spaces. The scope is then removed, leaving the Quill guide in place. The guide is dilated and the Tenckhoff catheter on its stylet (as discussed above) is advanced through the guide. The guide is removed carefully, ensuring that the catheter does not come out, and the stylet is then removed from the catheter. Tunnel creation and skin closure are as described above.

9.1.2.4 Comparison of the Three Techniques

Safety is the major advantage of the surgical procedure. It is carried out under direct vision and thus omentectomy (if necessary) and correct positioning of the catheter are possible. This procedure can also place any type of catheter.

The major advantage of the percutaneous method is that it does not require an involved preparation or operating room. The procedure is quick, relatively inexpensive, and, with an experienced operator (usually a nephrologist), the risk of complication is low. The incidence of fluid leak around the catheter is particularly low with this technique, even when the catheter is used immediately, as long as the infusion volumes are low during the first few weeks. Leakage is lower, the healing is faster, and, in experienced hands, overall outcome is better by this technique.

The advantages of the peritoneoscopy are that it can be done by the nephrologist, and that adhesions can be avoided under direct vision. The disadvantage of the percutaneous method is the potential for complications (including injury to viscera or bleeding), whereas the cost of the surgical technique and the initial expense of the peritoneoscope are the disadvantages of the latter two techniques. Fluid leaks are more common and healing takes longer following the surgical technique.

9.1.2.5 Postoperative Complications

Many of these are complications that are experienced with any surgical procedure, including trauma to an abdominal organ (most commonly the bowel) or to vessels, bleeding, infection, and bowel perforation. Specific complications are discussed below and in Table 9.3 [1]:

- Leakage around the catheter: This is more commonly seen in obese patients, and if the catheter is inserted through an incision (surgical) rather than through a puncture (percutaneous technique) wound of the peritoneal membrane. This usually represents nonhealing of the deeper wound through which the fluid is leaking. Once it occurs, the fluid amount should be reduced to lower intra-abdominal pressure, and sufficient time for healing should be given. If a patient is receiving CAPD, switching to nightly dialysis in a supine position and using less fill volume will help the healing process. The abdomen should be left empty during the daytime until the healing occurs and leakage stops.

Table 9.3 Common postoperative complications and their management

Complication	Management
Fluid leak	Decrease inflow volume Switch to cycler PD in supine position Keep abdomen empty when upright
Outflow problems	For supine patient, change positions Administer enema to move bowel loops Increase the vertical distance between the abdomen and the outflow bag
Tunnel infection	(1) Systemic antibiotics (2) If these fail or infection recurs, change the catheter and use a fresh site for the tunnel
Pain during dialysate flow	
• At the beginning of inflow, improving slowly. Ensure fluid is neither too hot nor too cold and exclude peritonitis	Usually reaction to acidic pH; raise the pH of dialysate;
• At the end of inflow	Reposition catheter;
• At the epigastrium (pulling of omentum)	Reposition catheter;
Cuff erosion	
• Partial	Good exit site care, leave the cuff alone
• Complete	Cuff can be carefully shaved off
Hernias and hemorrhoids	Reduce intra-abdominal pressure by decreasing inflow volume, switching to cycler PD in supine position

PD peritoneal dialysis

- Outflow problem: This is perhaps the most common and frustrating problem, manifesting as a decreased return of infused volume and leading to retention of fluid in the peritoneal cavity. Several steps can be taken to improve outflow. If constipation or decreased bowel movement is suspected, a laxative or a saline enema may be helpful in normalizing outflow (about 50% of outflow problems respond). The height of the bed from the outflow bag should be checked and increased to improve the gravitational pull. Other causes of outflow problems include mechanical obstruction, such as a clamp being left on, or the kinking/accidental suture of the catheter. If fibrin is observed in the outflow, 100–500 U heparin/l should be added to the dialysate. Although heparin appears to be helpful in preventing the problem, once the fibrin has blocked the catheter, heparin is of no use. Thus, in all new catheters and in the presence of peritonitis (which causes increased depositing of fibrin), heparin should be used. If the catheter is blocked by a fibrin plug, urokinase or tPA may be used in an attempt to dissolve the fibrin plug. Urokinase 5,000 IU is diluted with 0.9% saline solution to 40 ml. This volume is infused into the catheter and the catheter is clamped for 30–90 min. At the end of this time, the catheter is unclamped and the fluid drained out. If the treatment is unsuccessful, the procedure should be repeated with a higher dose of urokinase (10,000 IU diluted to 40 ml with 0.9% saline). Tissue plasminogen activator (TPA) can also be used. A 1 mg/ml TPA concentration is infused and left for 1–2 h, and has been reported to open up plugged PD catheters. More diluted solution of TPA in 10 ml of 0.9 saline can be used and 0.1 mg/ml strength has been reported to be effective. If the outflow problem is due to noncorrectable mechanical obstruction or due to incorrect positioning of the catheter tip, the catheter may have to be repositioned or replaced.

Exit infection: Presence of redness, pus, or discharge at the exit site should be treated promptly because infection may if untreated may involve cuff and tunnel any discharge should be cultured. First, the area must be cleaned thoroughly and a local antibacterial agent (such as povodine–iodine) applied at least once a day. Local treatment alone tends to be effective but, if not, a systemic antibiotic should be used. If the cuff is not involved (the skin over the cuff is not inflamed, and squeezing on the cuff produces no discharge or pus), infection of the exit site can be treated successfully without removal of the catheter.

Tunnel infection: Redness, pain, swelling, and induration over the tunnel are signs of tunnel infection. By squeezing the exit cuff, if purulent material is seen coming out of exit, it means that the cuff is involved and the infection is very difficult to treat. These infections do not usually respond to therapy, and the risk of recurrent peritonitis is high. If the infection does not respond to treatment, the catheter should be removed or replaced through a newly created tunnel, and antibiotic therapy should be continued for at least 1 week.

Pain with inflow: Timing of pain may be helpful in identifying the cause (see Table 9.3). Pain that is felt as soon as fluid inflows and that improves with time is likely to be due to the acidic pH of the fluid and can be corrected by increasing the pH. If the fluid is too cold or too warm, the patient may feel a similar type of pain. Pain occurring toward the end of inflow and worsening during the end of outflow is seen usually in the presence of peritonitis. Other causes of pain include adhesions, pull on the omentum (the pain is usually felt mainly in the epigastrium), and the catheter tip rubbing against the rectum or other viscera.

Cuff erosion: This tends to be the result of a tunnel being too short for the tunnel segment of the catheter, which, over time, forces the superficial cuff out. The extruded cuff can be carefully shaved off and the catheter left in place but the patient must be monitored carefully for any sign of infection.

Back pain: This is seen frequently in patients undergoing CAPD and requires that the patient be evaluated for other medical problems affecting the back. Changing to nighttime (supine) dialysis may relieve symptoms.

Hernias and hemorrhoids: Increased intra-abdominal pressure can cause abdominal hernia (particularly in children) and hemorrhoids. Decreasing the intra-abdominal pressure by decreasing volume in a nightly dialysis program may be helpful.

Peritonitis: This is discussed in Chapter 10.

9.2 Peritoneal Dialysis Fluid

This solution (the composition of which is given in Table 9.4) is dispensed in plastic bags that are larger in volume than the solution volume. In the USA, the basic anion is lactate and the pH of the commercially available solution is about 5.5 (to prevent caramelization of dextrose during sterilization). If a patient cannot tolerate this low pH, an alkali can be added to the solution but it is important that the pH is checked to prevent alkalinization of the solution. Sterile, pyrogen-free sodium hydroxide has been used for this purpose.

Bicarbonate solutions: Instead of lactate, bicarbonate solution or bicarbonate/lactate solutions are now available. A two-compartment bag keeps the bicarbonate solution separate from the rest of electrolytes, including calcium and magnesium, to avoid precipitation of their carbonate salts. Prior to use, the two solutions are mixed and infused. The bicarbonate solution has a higher pH and initial results are very encouraging. Harmful, long-term effects of an acidic dialysis fluid (lactate based) on the peritoneal membrane and on the function of leukocytes and macrophages have been reported but bicarbonate-based solutions have not been used at a large scale to fully asses the benefits.

9.2.1 Osmotic Agents

9.2.1.1 Dextrose

Glucose or dextrose are the osmotic agents that have traditionally been used in PD solutions. In comparison to glucose, the amount of anhydrous dextrose is lower for the corresponding solutions (e.g., 1.5% solution contains 1.36 g/dl of dextrose or 1.5 g/dl of glucose). UF rates depends on the concentration of the dextrose in the solution and duration of dwell in the peritoneal cavity. Thus a 1.5% dextrose solution left for over 3 hours will have very little or no net UF, while a 4.25%

Table 9.4 Composition of peritoneal dialysis fluid

Electrolytes	Standard solution (mEq/l)
Sodium	132
Potassium	0*
Calcium	2.5, 3.5
Magnesium	0.5, 1.5
Chloride	96–102
Lactate	35–40
Glucose (g/dl)**	1.5, 2.5, 3.5, 4.25
pH	5.2–5.5

* Potassium is often added to maintain serum concentration in normal range.
** Dextrose is usually used as the osmotic agent; being anhydrous, a corresponding concentration is given by a smaller weight than glucose.

dextrose solution left for 6 hours or longer may still have significant net UF. After reaching a peak UF rate at a dwell time of 2–3 h, plasma and dialysate osmolarity equilibrates and the UF rate slows [2]. This is followed by a gradual absorption of the intraperitoneal fluid across the peritoneal membrane and lymphatics. The dissipation of osmolarity is mainly a result of the absorption of glucose from the peritoneal cavity. It is proposed that the net glucose uptake (GU) is related to the glucose concentration and is predicted by the following formula [3]:

$$GU(g/day) = (11.3 \times [G] - 10.9) \times V$$

Where G = average daily dialysate glucose concentration and V = dialysate inflow volume (l/day).

Normal glucose uptake ranges from 100–300 g/day in CAPD patients, depending on the glucose concentration of the solution used. Thus, the patient may get as much as 1,200 calories per day from the dextrose in the dialysate. The long-term deleterious effects of dextrose and the products of its degradation (as a result of lower pH of the solution) on peritoneal membrane are a source of ongoing discussions [3].

The UF volume is dependent on three major factors:

Dialysate dextrose concentration (osmolarity)
Dwell time
Peritoneal membrane characteristics

There is wide variation in the rate of absorption of glucose; faster glucose absorption with a longer dwell time reduces the net UF volume, even with 4.25% dextrose solutions. This is discussed later, under the section on membrane transport characteristics.

9.2.1.2 Alternative Agents

Several osmotic agents other than glucose have been tried with varying degrees of success. These are listed in Table 9.5.

Amino Acid Solutions

Amino acid solutions have been studied as an alternative. In general, these have UFR that are similar to that of glucose; thus, a 1% amino acid solution is equivalent to 1.5% dextrose in terms of UF volume, and a 2.0–2.76% amino acid solution is equivalent to 4.25% dextrose. Amino acids tend, however, to be absorbed faster and with longer dwell times (8 h or more), the UF volume is often lower than with dextrose solution. There is some indication that amino acids may increase the permeability of the membrane for creatinine by about 10%. Their beneficial nutritional effect is controversial, and with older, unselected amino acid solutions, there did not seem to be any significant benefit. Recent studies using more essential amino acids and

Table 9.5 Alternative osmotic agents to glucose and their potential complications (Reproduced from [4]. With permission)

Osmotic agents	Potential complications
Gelatin	Prolonged half-life and immunogenicity of some preparations
Xylitol	Peritoneal pain, lactic acidosis, hyperuricemia, carcinogenicity, and deterioration of liver function
Sorbitol	Metabolized via polyol pathway, which may aggravate neuropathy, lactic acidosis, hyperuricemia, and hyperosmolarity
Mannitol	Lactic acidosis, hyperuricemia
Fructose	Metabolized via polyol pathway, which may aggravate neuropathy, hypernatremia, lactic acidosis, hyperuricemia, and hypertriglyceridemia
Dextrans	Risk of bleeding and systemic absorption
Polyanions	Damage to peritoneum, cardiovascular instability
Amino acids	Increased concentration of nitrogenous products in blood, increased hydrogen ion generation, expensive, optimal formulation not yet determined, difficult to sterilize in combination with glucose, and nonphysiological high plasma levels of amino acids
Glycerol	Retention, hypertriglyceridemia, sterile peritonitis, greater ultrafiltration than glucose but of short duration, resulting in low net ultrafiltration capacity, and hyperosmolality
Glucose polymers	Prolonged half-life, impaired metabolism in uremia, accumulation of maltose, and potential for high caloric loads

less non-essential amino acids (mainly glycine and alanine) have, however, shown some beneficial effects in patients with protein malnutrition [5]. These are usually used once a day, with more frequent use there is risk of metabolic acidosis and an increase in urea concentration is seen.

Icodextrin Solution

Icodextrin is a glucose polymer that is derived from starch, containing many glucose units bonded together. In the peritoneal cavity, it slowly breaks down into smaller units thus causing sustained osmolarity and UF. This is particularly helpful in high transporters in removing fluid, especially during the long dwell time (>6 h). Thus, in CCPD (Automated PD, APD) patients, icodextrin solutions can be used during the daytime and in CAPD patients during the night dwell to achieve adequate UF. Higher blood levels of maltose and maltotriose have been observed with its use, this level interferes with the glucose assay by the glucose dehydrogenase pyroquinolone quinine method. The assay measures both glucose and malose thus giving false high readings. Patients using icodextrin must not use this blood glucose assay.

9.3 Delivery Mechanism

Delivery of fluid from the source to the peritoneal catheter is usually accomplished by using a transfer set, of which, two main types are in common use:

Straight transfer sets: This comprises a straight piece of tubing, one end of which is connected to the catheter, the other end to the PD bags (for CAPD). The patient connects a full bag, opens the clamps, and instills the fluid into the abdominal cavity, rolls up the empty bag and transfer set, and carries it with them. At the end of the dwell time, the patient unrolls the empty bag, drains the fluid out into this bag, disconnects and discards the bag, connects a new full bag, and repeats the process. The transfer sets are changed periodically (once every few months).

Y Sets: This comprises a Y tube with one empty and one full bag connected to the two arms of the Y and the third arm connected to an extension tube that is connected to the catheter. This configuration allows patients to disconnect and remove the empty bag (see Fig. 9.4). Use of the Y-set with a flush before the peritoneal fill (inflow) has been reported to decrease the incidence of peritonitis.

9.4 Peritoneal Dialysis Techniques

All the techniques are graphically described in Fig. 9.5.

9.4.1 Continuous Ambulatory Peritoneal Dialysis (CAPD)

This requires only connecting tubes and bags of solutions (usually 2 L of solution in 3-L bags), using gravity to fill and empty the peritoneal cavity. The most commonly used method uses four exchanges per day, but, in some patients, five exchanges are necessary. A small number of patients use three exchanges, but this is inadequate under most circumstances, and should be discouraged.

9.4.2 Automated Peritoneal Dialysis (APD)

This technique uses a cycler with or without added manual exchanges. The two forms are continuous cycling PD (CCPD) and nocturnal intermittent PD (NIPD). In CCPD, at night, a cycler is used to have a few automated exchanges and, during daytime, there are one or two manual exchanges. The NIPD involves automated nightly exchanges and during the daytime the peritoneal cavity remains empty. There are different variations of APD with a variety of dwell times. Tidal PD (TPD) is also a variant of APD. All of these techniques are graphically shown in Fig. 9.5. In this technique, the patient loads the bags of solution on to a cycler and connects the catheter to this cycler just before going to sleep. During the night, the cycler makes

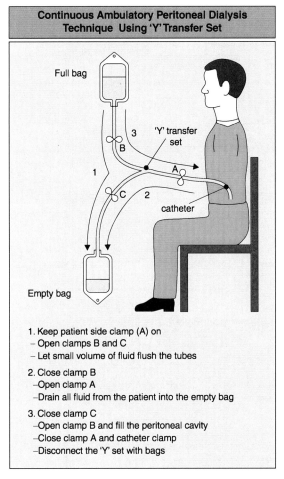

Fig. 9.4 Continuous ambulatory peritoneal dialysis technique using a "Y" transfer set

four to five or more exchanges automatically. In the morning, 2 L of solution are left in the abdomen and the patient disconnects from the cycler. During the day, there is usually no exchange and, at night, the procedure is repeated. Sometimes, to improve clearance, an additional exchange is performed in the early evening or late afternoon.

9.4.2.1 Tidal Peritoneal Dialysis (TPD)

In an attempt to better use the time during inflow and outflow, when the peritoneal cavity may be empty without any dialysis, the TPD technique was developed. The peritoneal cavity is filled to the maximum capacity tolerable and, after a relatively short dwell time (e.g., 20 min), half of the volume is drained out and replaced. This is

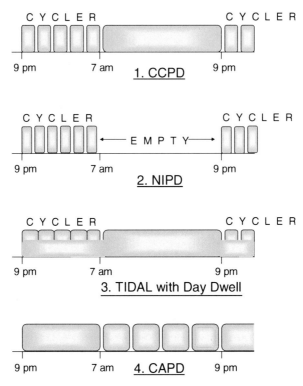

Fig. 9.5 Different types of peritoneal dialysis techniques. The *yellow box* represents the peritoneal cavity filled with fluid, each box representing one exchange

repeated (at equal intervals), ensuring ongoing dialysis and assuring that the cavity is never empty. The cost of the large volume of fluid needed for this technique is high, the persistently high intra-abdominal pressure can increase the risk of certain complications (such as hernias of the viscera), UF calculations are more complex, and a specialized cycler is needed for this technique. It is more frequently used in children.

9.4.2.2 Cyclers

Several different versions of these simple machines are available commercially, each of which allows the desired volume of fluid to flow into the abdomen automatically. After the set dwell time, the machine permits the outflow to begin and measures the outflow volume. It also tracks the difference between the inflow and outflow, thus measuring the UF volume. Opening and closing of different sets of clamps performs the alternate cycling. The cyclers also warm the dialysate and can repeat outflow if the desired volume has not been recovered. Failure to provide an appropriate volume of inflow or outflow can trigger alarms and shut off the machine.

References

1. Tenckhoff H. *Peritoneal Dialysis Manual*. Washington, DC: University of Washington; 1974.
2. Twardowski ZJ, Khanna R, Nolph KD. Osmotic agents and ultrafiltration in peritoneal dialysis. *Nephron* 1986, 42:93–101.
3. Feriani M, Ronco C, La Greca G. Solutions for peritoneal dialysis. In *Replacement of renal function by dialysis. 4th Edition*. Edited by C Jacobs, CM Kjellstrand, KM Koch and JF Winchester. Dordrecht: Kluwer Academic Publications, 1996:520–546.
4. Diaz-Buxo JA. Clinical use of peritoneal dialysis. In *Clinical Dialysis*, 3rd edition. Edited by AR Nissenson, RN Fine and DE Gentile. Norwalk: Appleton and Lange, 1995:376–425.
5. Jones MR, Martis L, Algrim CE et al. Amino acids solutions for CAPD: rationale and clinical experience. *Miner Electrolyte Metab* 1992, 18:309–315.

Chapter 10
Dose of Peritoneal Dialysis

The dose of peritoneal dialysis (PD) has traditionally been measured by small solute (urea and creatinine) clearances. However, based on one large study from Mexico (Adequacy of Peritoneal Dialysis in Mexico [ADEMEX]) and a small study from Hong Kong, Kidney Disease Outcomes Quality Initiative (KDOQI) guidelines have been modified to a lower target of Kt/V_{urea} (K is the plasma urea clearance, t is the duration of dialysis, and V_{urea} is the volume of distribution of urea), and creatinine clearance as a dose measure has been omitted. However, a previous study from North America (Canada–USA [CANUSA]) had suggested the previously held higher targets. Several studies have shown that the outcome in these patients is directly dependent on the residual renal function rather than peritoneal clearance. In the opinion of this author, from our experience with intermittent peritoneal dialysis (IPD), we must be very vigilant about the dose of dialysis and must not reduce our target values based on two studies from populations that are smaller in size and have a different nutritional intake. Recognizing this, the European Guideline, while reducing the target, recommends that only the contribution made by the peritoneal membrane should be considered in measuring the dose, and renal clearance should not be added. The prognosis of PD patients is influenced directly by the dose of dialysis. Because the contribution of residual renal function to the total dialysis dose is significant, it is important that renal contribution and the total dose of dialysis are both measured frequently. If either of these decrease significantly, the patient must be monitored very closely and, at the first sign of under-dialysis, therapy must be modified to avoid premature death from under-dialysis. Because of these concerns, this section will discuss the traditional methods and targets [1].

10.1 Weekly Creatinine Clearance

Boen et al. [2] were the first to propose that weekly creatinine clearance (WClCr) be used to quantify dialysis dose. Total WClCr combines the glomerular filtration rate (GFR) with the peritoneal creatinine clearance (WpClCr) and normalizes it for a body surface area (BSA) of $1.73 \, m^2$:

S. Ahmad, *Manual of Clinical Dialysis*, DOI 10.1007/978-0-387-09651-3_10,
© Springer Science+Business Media LLC 2009

1. Calculate residual GFR, convert it to weekly clearance
2. Calculate peritoneal creatinine clearance and convert it to weekly clearance (WpClCr)
3. Estimate BSA from height and weight
4. Normalize the WpClCr to a BSA of $1.73\,m^2$
5. Weekly creatinine clearance = GFR (from Step 1) + WpClCr per $1.73\,m^2$ (from Step 5)

10.1.1 Residual Glomerular Filtration Rate

With declining GFR, the tubular secretion of creatinine increases; creatinine clearance overestimates true GFR. To correct for the tubular creatinine secretion, the average of urea and creatinine clearance is used to estimate GFR.

$$GFR = (\text{renal urea clearance} + \text{renal creatinine clearance})/2$$

Some investigators use 50% of measured creatinine clearance as GFR, thus, GFR = 0.5 renal creatinine clearance. The first method is more commonly used.

Example

A 70-kg, 140-cm tall, 45-year-old man is on continuous ambulatory PD (CAPD), four exchanges/day, each using 2 L of fluid. Twenty-four-hour urine collection and blood values are:

Urine volume, 90 ml; urine creatinine, 140 mg/dl; serum creatinine, 9 mg/dl; urine urea, 650 mg/dl; BUN, 80 mg/dl.
GFR calculation (using formula UV/p):
Renal creatinine clearance (rClCr) = 9.7 ml/min

(At this level of renal impairment, a significant part of the creatinine is secreted by the renal tubules, thus, only a fraction of 9.7 ml/min is a result of glomerular filtration).

Renal urea clearance (rClU) = 5.07 ml/min
GFR = $(5.07 + 9.7)/2 = 7.4$ ml/min; 10,080 min/week = 74.5 L/week

10.1.2 Peritoneal Creatinine Clearance

Peritoneal creatinine clearance (pClCr) is measured by collecting all peritoneal outflow for 24 h and measuring creatinine in the dialysate and in the blood. The usual clearance formula is used.

Example

The above patient collects all four exchanges in 24 h and the total volume is 10 L, the creatinine concentration in the dialysate is 8.0 mg/dl, and serum creatinine is still 9 mg/dl. Thus:

$$\text{pClCr} = (8\,\text{mg/dl} \times 10,000\,\text{ml})/(9\,\text{mg/dl} \times 1440\,\text{min})$$
$$= 6.1\,\text{ml/min or } 6.1\,\text{ml/min} \times 10080\,\text{min/week} = 61.5\,\text{L/week}$$

10.1.3 Correction for Body Surface Area

The WClCr should be normalized for $1.73\,\text{m}^2$. BSA from weight (kilograms) and height (centimeters) can be either estimated on a nomogram (see Fig. 10.1) [3], or calculated by one of the following formulae [1]:

DuBois and DuBois method: BSA $(\text{m}^2) = 71.84 \times \text{weight}^{0.425} \times \text{height}^{0.725}$
Gehan and George method: BSA $(\text{m}^2) = 0.0235 \times \text{weight}^{0.51456} \times \text{height}^{0.42246}$
Haycock method: BSA $(\text{m}^2) = 0.024265 \times \text{weight}^{0.5378} \times \text{height}^{0.3964}$

Often the desired (ideal) weight rather than actual weight is used to calculate BSA, this is to reduce the effect of malnourished or obese weight.

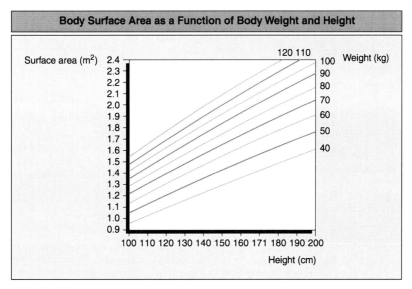

Fig. 10.1 Body surface area as a function of body weight and height. Reproduced from [3] with permission

10.1.4 Total Weekly Creatinine Clearance Calculation

For the patient in the example, the BSA $= 1.57\,m^2$ and, thus:
   WpClCr $= (61.5\,L/week/1.57\,m^2)$ or $67.7\,L/week/1.73\,m^2$ $(61.51\times 1.73/1.57)$.

From the above, we can therefore calculate that the (BSA-corrected) total WClCr is: total WClCr$/1.73\,m^2 = 74.5\,l/week(residualGFR) + 67.7\,L/week(pClCr, BSA - corrected) = 142.2\,l/week/1.73\,m^2$.

It is important to note that 74.5 l of the 142.2 l is contributed by the residual GFR and as this declines, the overall uremia control will become less effective. In summary, the steps to calculate weekly creatinine clearance are: collect peritoneal dialysate outflow for 24 h, measure volume (dV), creatinine (dCr), urea (for Kt/V calculation), and serum creatinine and blood urea nitrogen (BUN). Collect urine for 24 h, measure volume (uV), creatinine (uCr), and urea (uU). Perform calculations, as detailed above.

10.2 Urea Clearance Concept (Kt/V_{urea})

The second method of calculating dialysis dose is by the use of the urea kinetics concept. A combination of peritoneal and renal urea clearances, relative to the volume of distribution of urea, give a value of total Kt/V_{urea}.

10.2.1 Volume of Distribution of Urea

The volume of distribution of urea (V_{urea}) is equivalent to the total body water (TBW) and can be estimated by several methods.

1. Direct estimation from weight: Normally, water represents 58% of body weight. Thus, the total body water $= 0.58 \times$ weight ($0.58 \times 70\,kg$ in our patient $= 40.6\,L$).This method is not very accurate, because sex and age also have an effect on the water fraction of the body weight.
2. Use of specific formulae: One of three formulae can be used to calculate body weight—the first two are used in adults and the last in children [1].
   Watson Formula.
   For men: V (total body water in liters) $= 2.447 + 0.3362 \times$ weight (kg) $+ 0.174 \times$ height (cm) $0.09516 \times$ age (years).
   For women: V (total body water in liters) $= 2.097 + 0.2466 \times$ weight $+ 0.1069 \times$ height
   Hume Formula:
   For men: V (l) $= 14.012934 + 0.296785 \times$ weight $+ 0.192786 \times$ height.
   For women: V (l) $= 35.270121 + 0.183809 \times$ weight $+ 0.344547 \times$ height

Mellits–Cheek Formula for Children:
For boys: V (when height < 132.7 cm) $= -1.927 + 0.465 \times$ weight $+ 0.045 \times$ height; V (when height > 132.7 cm) $= -21.993 + 0.406 \times$ weight $+ 0.209 \times$ height.
For girls: V (when height < 110.8 cm) $= -0.076 + 0.507 \times$ weight $+ 0.013 \times$ height; V (when height > 110.8 cm) $= -10.313 + 0.252 \times$ weight $+ 0.154 \times$ height

Example

1. Calculate the volume of distribution of urea (V_{urea}): From the Watson method, the V_{urea} for the patient described in Section 10.2.1 $= 36.7$ L
2. Calculate the peritoneal urea clearance (pCl_{urea}) : $pCl_{urea} = 10$ L/day (dialysate urea $=$ serum urea, then clearance $=$ dialysate flow rate)
3. Calculate the weekly peritoneal urea clearance ($WpCl_{urea}$, pKt) $= 10$ L/day $\times 7$ days/week $= 70$ L/week

Weekly peritoneal $Kt/V_{urea} = 70$ L/36.7 $\times$ L $= 1.9$ L.
Weekly renal urea clearance $= 5.07$ ml/min $\times 10,080$ min/week $= 51.1 \times$ L/week.
Weekly renal Kt/V $= 51.1 \times$ L/36.7 $\times$ L $= 1.39$.
Total weekly $Kt/V_{urea} = 1.91 + 1.39 = 3.3$.
Note that without the renal contribution, the total weekly Kt/V_{urea} is only $1.91 \times$ L.

10.3 Recommended Dose of Dialysis

Based on several outcome studies, the following recommendations for the minimum dose of dialysis have been made by the old National Kidney Foundation (NKF)– DOQI guidelines [1]:

Dialysis dose should be measured in terms of both:
Weekly total creatinine clearance
Weekly total Kt/V_{urea}
The minimum dialysis dose:

For CAPD:

Weekly total creatinine clearance > 60 l/week/1.73 m^2
Weekly total $Kt/V_{urea} > 2.0$

For continuous cycling PD (CCPD):

Weekly creatinine clearance > 63 l/week/1.73 m^2
Weekly $Kt/V_{urea} > 2.1$

For nocturnal intermittent PD (NIPD):

Weekly creatinine clearance $> 66 \text{l/week} / 1.73 \text{ m}^2$
Weekly $Kt/V_{urea} > 2.2$

Current KDOQI guideline: As discussed above, the current guideline has made some changes in recommendations:

Guideline 2: Solute Clearance Targets and Measurements:

2.1 For patients with residual kidney function (RKF) (considered to be significant when urine volume is $> 100 \text{ mL/d}$):
2.1.1 The minimal "delivered" dose of total small-solute clearance should be a total (peritoneal and kidney) Kt/V_{urea} of at least 1.7 per week.
2.1.2 Total solute clearance (residual kidney and peritoneal, in terms of Kt/V_{urea}) should be measured within the first month after initiating dialysis therapy and at least once every 4 months thereafter.
2.1.3 If the patient has greater than 100 mL/d of residual kidney volume and residual kidney clearance is being considered as part of the patient's total weekly solute clearance goal, a 24-hour urine collection for urine volume and solute clearance determinations should be obtained at a minimum of every 2 months.
2.2 For patients without RKF (urine volume is $< 100 \text{ mL/d}$):
2.2.1 The minimal "delivered" dose of total small-solute clearance should be a peritoneal Kt/V_{urea} of at least 1.7 per week measured within the first month after starting dialysis therapy and at least once every 4 months thereafter.

Thus, the new guideline does not recommend creatinine clearance measurement and the weekly Kt/V_{urea} minimum target has been reduced to 1.7. **The new guideline also does not recommend different targets for different forms of the peritoneal dialysis techniques. However, because of concerns about under-dialysis, this chapter would leave the old recommendations and targets.**

10.3.1 Potential Problem with Dose Measurements

Malnourished patients with muscle wasting will have lower than ideal body weight. This leads to lower calculated V and overestimation of Kt/V. In such cases, the V_{urea} determination should be calculated using the desired weight rather than the current body weight.

10.3.2 Frequency of Dose Determination

The new NKF–DOQI guidelines recommend that the dose in terms of "total solute clearance (residual kidney and peritoneal, in terms of Kt/V_{urea}) should be measured within the first month after initiating dialysis therapy and at least once every 4 months thereafter. However if the patient has greater than 100 mL/d of residual urine volume and residual kidney clearance is being considered as part of the patient's total weekly solute clearance goal, a 24-hour urine collection for urine volume and solute clearance determinations should be obtained at a minimum of every 2 months."

10.4 Peritoneal Function Test

Wide interpatient variability in solute and solvent movement across the peritoneal membrane has long been observed, and the ultrafiltration (UF) rate has been known to change over time in the same patient. Twardowski et al. [4] first described a peritoneal equilibration test (PET) to assess the peritoneal function in terms of the rate of solute transport. A subsequent study showed the prognostic value of the PET and led to increased interest in use of this test [5]. It is now routinely used to monitor membrane function in both new and established patients.

10.4.1 Traditional Peritoneal Equilibration Test

A 2 L volume of 2.5% dextrose solution is instilled in an empty peritoneal cavity and dialysate samples are obtained at 0, 2, and 4 h to measure creatinine and glucose concentrations. At the end of the 4-h dwell time, all of the fluid is drained out, the total volume is measured, and the sample volumes (drawn during the 2 and 4 h) are added to the final volume. A blood sample is also obtained at 4 h to measure serum creatinine. Two curves are then plotted. One curve plots the 0-, 2-, and 4-h values of dextrose in the dialysate outflow as a fraction of the initial dialysate dextrose concentration (D/D_0). The second curve plots the ratio of dialysate to plasma creatinine concentrations $(D/P_{creatinine})$ (see Fig. 10.2) [6].

10.4.2 Fast Peritoneal Equilibration Test

The fast PET is a simpler and less expensive version of the traditional equilibration test and is initiated by the patient at home. After emptying the peritoneal cavity completely, the patient instills 2 L of 2.5% dextrose solution and arrives at the clinic within 4 h. At 4 h, the fluid is drained out completely, the volume is measured, and blood and dialysate samples are sent for measurement of dextrose and creatinine concentrations. The excellent reproducibility of this test makes it a useful tool.

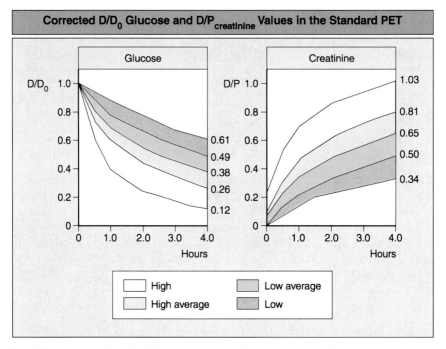

Fig. 10.2 Range of values for D/D_0 glucose and $D/P_{creatinine}$ (corrected) in standard peritoneal equilibration test (PET). *D* dialysate concentration, *P* plasma concentration, D_0 dialysate concentration at time $= 0$ (reproduced from [6] with permission)

Table 10.1 Transport characteristics of fast 4-h peritoneal equilibration test

Transport type	$D/P_{creatinine}$	Dextrose (D/D_0)	Net ultrafiltration (ml)
High (hi)	0.82–1.03	0.092–0.25	30–400
High-average (ha)	0.66–0.81	0.26–0.37	31–350
Mean	0.65	0.38	350
Low-average (la)	0.50–0.64	0.39–0.48	350–600
Low (lo)	0.34–0.49	0.49–0.61	600–1275

D dialysate concentration, *P* plasma concentration, D_0 dialysate concentration at time $= 0$

10.4.3 Results of the Peritoneal Equilibration Test

The peritoneal membrane can be characterized as either a high, average, or low transporter, on the basis of UF volume data, $D/P_{creatinine}$, and D/D_0 dextrose. Four groups of patients have been characterized according to their 4-h results; high, high average, low average, or low transporters. Each subgroup is separated from the next one by a value of one standard deviation. The average values at 4 h are a $D/P_{creatinine}$ ratio of 0.65, a D/D_0 value of 0.29, and net UF of 320 ml (see Table 10.1). Patients

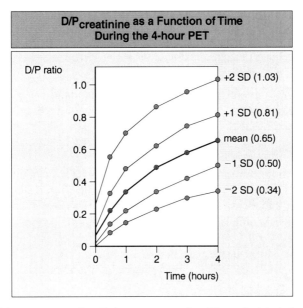

Fig. 10.3 *D* dialysate concentration, *P* plasma concentration, *SD* standard deviation (adapted from [7] with permission)

with high transport characteristics have a faster dissipation of dextrose, a lower net UF rate (see Fig. 10.3) [7], and higher $^{D/P}$creatinine ^{values}.

10.5 Use of Fast Peritoneal Equilibration Test Results in Selecting a Peritoneal Dialysis Regimen

The PET results are useful in assessing membrane function and in deciding which form of PD is most suitable for the patient. Thus, a high transporter will have faster dissipation of dextrose and a longer dwell time of CAPD would lead to a lower net UF and an inability to control fluid excess. In a low–average transporter, rapid exchanges will not remove enough solute and will lead to wastage of dialysate. Thus, a high transporter will benefit from a shorter dwell time of cycler-assisted dialysis, whereas for those with lower transport, CAPD might be a better choice. It must be stressed that PET does not give information on adequacy of dialysis; adequacy must be assessed by calculation of Kt/V_{urea} and weekly creatinine clearance (see above). In a cross-sectional study, the D/P_{urea} values in a 24 h collection for all four transporter groups were 0.95 [8]. The 4-h ratios were 1.0, 0.92, 0.85, and 0.75 for high, high average, low average, and low transporters, respectively.

10.5.1 Selection of Technique

Four major considerations in selection of the technique are:

1. Patient preference, life style, and practical considerations: Patients with limited time during daytime for exchanges, those for whom physical appearance is important, and those with good social support at home usually prefer a variant of automated peritoneal dialysis (APD). On the other hand, those who dislike being tied to a machine, are unable to sleep with cycler, or who have limited support at home may prefer CAPD.
2. Medical considerations: A particular technique may provide optimal solute clearance or fluid control. Thus, the selection may be APD with short exchanges to increase the solute clearance. However, shorter dwell may increase free water loss relative to sodium loss causing hypernatremia. If potential for peritonitis increases, APD with less connect/disconnect may be preferable over CAPD.
3. PET considerations: In the past, the impact of the PET was overestimated and the criteria for technique choices were too rigid. These are now considered to be less important.
4. Cost considerations: The cost of fluid and cycler should not be a more important consideration than patient preference and medical considerations.

10.5.1.1 Empirical Approach to Deciding a Peritoneal Dialysis Regimen

The following empirical approach can be used to start patients on some form of PD therapy; however, the dose of dialysis must be monitored regularly and adjusted as necessary [1].

Patients with GFR $> 2\,\text{ml}/\text{min}$:

For CAPD: BSA $< 1.7\,\text{m}^2$: $2\text{L}\times$ four exchanges/day; BSA $1.7\text{--}2.0\,\text{m}^2$: $2.5\text{L}\times$ four exchanges/day; BSA $> 2.0\,\text{m}^2$: $3.0\text{L}\times$ four exchanges/day
For CCPD: BSA $< 1.7\,\text{m}^2$: $2\text{L}\times$ four exchanges (9 h/night) $+2\text{L}/\text{day}$; BSA $1.7\text{--}2.0\,\text{m}^2$: $2.5\text{L}\times$ four exchanges (9 h/night)$+2\text{L}/\text{day}$BSA $> 2.0\,\text{m}^2$: $3.0\text{L}\times$ four exchanges (9 h/night) $+2\text{L}/\text{day}$

Patients with GFR $< 2\,\text{ml}/\text{min}$:

For CAPD: BSA $< 1.7\,\text{m}^2$: $2.5\text{L}\times$ four exchanges /day; BSA $1.7\text{--}2.0\,\text{m}^2$: $3.0\text{L}\times$ four exchanges/day; BSA $> 2.0\,\text{m}^2$: $3.0\text{L}\times$ four exchanges/day (added exchange at night should be considered)
For CCPD: BSA $< 1.7\,\text{m}^2$: $2.5\text{L}\times$ four exchanges (9 h /night) $+2\text{L}/\text{day}$; BSA $1.7\text{--}2.0\,\text{m}^2$: $3.0\text{L}\times$ four exchanges (9 h/night) $+2.5$ L/day; BSA $> 2.0\,\text{m}^2$: $3.0\text{L}\times$ 4 exchanges (10 h/night) $+3\text{L}\times$ two exchanges/day
For NIPD: The intermittent NIPD needs to be closely monitored for GFR changes and adequacy of dialysis as well as membrane functions, and the regimen must be modified accordingly.

References

1. Anonymous. NKF-DOQI Clinical practice guidelines for peritoneal dialysis adequacy. National Kidney Foundation-Dialysis Outcomes Quality Initiative. *Am J* Kidney Dis 1997, 30(Suppl 2):S67–S136.
2. Boen ST, Haagsma-Schouten WAG et al. Long-term peritoneal dialysis and a dialysis index. *Dial Transplant* 1978, 7:377.
3. Diaz-Buxo JA. Chronic peritoneal dialysis prescription. In *Handbook of Dialysis 2nd Edition.* Edited by JT Daugirdas and TS Ing. Philadelphia: Lippincott-Raven, 1993, pp. 310–327.
4. Twardowski ZJ. Clinical value of standardized equilibration tests in CAPD patients. *Blood Purif* 1989, 7:95–108.
5. Verger C, Larpent L, Dumontet M. Prognostic value of peritoneal equilibration curves in CAPD patients. In *Frontiers in Peritoneal Dialysis.* Edited by JF Maher and JF Winchester. New York: Rich and Associates, 1986, pp. 88–93.
6. Diaz-Buxo JA. Clinical use of peritoneal dialysis. In *Clinical Dialysis 2nd Edition.* Edited by AR Nissenson, RN Fine, and DE Gentile. Norwalk: Appleton and Lange, 1990, vol 13, pp. 256–300.
7. Twardowski ZJ et al. Peritoneal equilibration test. *Perit Dial Bull* 1987, 7:138–140.
8. Jensen RA, Nolph KD, Moore HL et al. Weight limitations for adequate therapy using commonly performed CAPD and IPD regimens. *Seminars Dial* 1994, 7:61.

Chapter 11
Complications of Peritoneal Dialysis

Table 11.1 lists the complications associated with peritoneal dialysis, some of which are discussed below.

11.1 Peritonitis

Historically, the use of peritoneal dialysis (PD) was restrained by the frequent occurrence of peritonitis. As the technique has improved, the infection rate has decreased considerably but it remains the most significant complication. In the USA, the time to first infection using a straight set is 11.4 months and with a Y-set it is 20.6 months [2]. This infection rate is higher with continuous ambulatory PD (CAPD) than was reported with intermittent peritoneal dialysis (IPD) or is presently observed with continuous cycling PD (CCPD). The difference probably reflects the increased number of connections and disconnections with CAPD in comparison with the other two techniques. Other factors associated with increased risk of infection include the *lower pH and higher osmolarity* of the dialysate, both of these can inhibit the macrophage and leukocyte ability to fight the microorganisms. Similarly, *the lower calcium* in the dialysate has been proposed to reduce the antimicrobial action of macrophages, thus, higher infection rates may be seen with 2.5 mEq/l calcium dialysate than with higher calcium dialysate. Patients with very low *levels of immunoglobulin G* have been reported to have more infections.

11.1.1 Clinical Diagnosis

The presence of any two of the following is sufficient for a clinical diagnosis of peritonitis:

– Clinical signs and symptoms of peritoneal inflammation (e.g., pain, discomfort, tenderness, rebound tenderness)

S. Ahmad, *Manual of Clinical Dialysis*, DOI 10.1007/978-0-387-09651-3_11,
© Springer Science+Business Media LLC 2009

Table 11.1 Complications of peritoneal dialysis

Complication	Cause	Corrective measures

Peritonitis
   Bacterial
   Fungal
   Chemical/sterile
	See Section 11.1	

Inadequate dialysis	See Section 11.3	
Exit site and tunnel infections	See Section 9.1.2.5	
Abdominal wall complications	Caused by the increased intra-abdominal pressure	Surgical correction, if needed

Hernias
   Umbilical
   Inguinal
   Incisional
(catheter sites)
   Epigastric
   Ventral
   Cystocele
   Others
		In recurring cases, decrease intra-abdominal pressure by changing to nocturnal intermittent peritoneal dialysis and keeping peritoneal cavity empty while upright

Genital edema (scrotal and labial)	Secondary to either a wall defect	Most leaks improve with rest insertion site Reduced pressure (see above)
Hydrothorax (pleural leak)	or a leak around the catheter	
Malnutrition	See Section 11.4	
Cardiovascular complications	See Section 11.6	
Sclerosing encapsulating peritonitis		
Back pain	Change in posture due to the presence of a large volume of fluid	Decrease pressure (see above) Regular exercise [1]
Intra-abdominal abscesses		
Hemoperitoneum	See Section 11.8 and Table 11.6 for causes	
Chyloperitoneum		

– Presence of cloudy outflow fluid, with a white blood cell (WBC) count > 100 and $>50\%$ neutrophils
– Presence of organism on Gram stain and/or on culture

Table 11.2 displays the clinical manifestations of peritonitis. A cloudy appearance of the peritoneal effluent, which often appears suddenly, is the most common sign of peritonitis, and may be a useful early warning sign. It is difficult to see through the bag wall and patients must be trained to put the bag against light and look for a cloudy appearance. It is important to note that cloudy fluid can also be caused by conditions other than infection (see Table 11.3) [3]. Measurement of total and differential cell counts is a useful clinical tool in the diagnosis of peritonitis. An

Table 11.2 Clinical manifestation of peritonitis

Presenting symptom and signs	Frequency of occurrence in peritonitis (%)
Symptoms	
Abdominal pain	80
Fever and chills	20–30
Nausea and vomiting	25
Diarrhea or constipation	10–15
Signs	
Cloudy effluent	>95
Abdominal tenderness	70
Rebound tenderness	50
Temperature >37.5°C	30–50
Bloody effluent	20

Table 11.3 Causes of cloudy peritoneal effluent.

Infectious peritonitis (most common cause)
Chemical peritonitis
Eosinophilic peritonitis
Blood in the peritoneum
Chyloperitoneum
Diarrhea
Inflammation of abdominal organs (e.g., appendicitis, pancreatitis, salpingitis)
Excessive fibrin production

infecting pathogen (bacteria) may be present for 24–48 h before the fluid clouds and the cell count increases, but an increase in cell count in excess of $50\,cells/mm^3$ is usually associated with infection. A differential count that shows neutrophils to make up >50% of the total cell number is even more sensitive and specific for peritonitis.

11.1.1.1 Clinical Work-Up of Suspected Peritonitis

After a careful history and examination, the peritoneal effluent should be sent for:

- Gram staining
- Total cell count and differential WBC count
- Culture and testing for antimicrobial sensitivity.

Gram stain of the peritoneal effluent is a valuable tool (although it is positive in only about one third of cases) and may be of help in identifying fungal infection. The microbial culture is the most important step in identifying the organism, deciding the appropriate therapy, and determining follow-up of the patients' progress. To maximize the chances of growing the infecting organism, at least 50 ml of effluent should be sent to the laboratory for concentration or filtration, after which the substrate can be cultured. A separate 10 ml of effluent should be cultured (in a minimum of two

Table 11.4 Common pathogenic organisms and the frequency of their involvement in peritonitis

Organism	Frequency of isolation (%)
Gram-positive bacteria	80–90
Staphylococcus epidermidis	
Staphylococcus aureus	30–40
Streptococcus viridans	5–10
Streptococcus faecalis	5–10
Gram-negative bacteria	
Escherichia coli	5–10
Klebsiella/Enterobacter spp.	5
Pseudomonas spp.	<10
Acinetobacter spp.	<5
Mycobacterium spp.	<5
Others	<5
Fungi	
Candida spp.	1–10
Other fungi	<5
Culture negative	5–20

blood culture bottles) and set aside to be subcultured when the medium becomes turbid. Determining antimicrobial sensitivity is an important part of the work-up.

Bacterial organisms cause 80–90% of peritonitis; staphylococci are the most common causal agents. Of the Gram-negative organisms, *Escherichia coli*, *Enterobacter*, *Klebsiella*, and *Pseudomonas* are the most frequently isolated. Fungal peritonitis is seen in <10% cases (see Table 11.4).

11.1.2 Therapy

11.1.2.1 Lavages

Treatment of suspected peritonitis should be started immediately after the necessary fluid samples have been obtained. Concern that the lower pH and higher osmolarity of the PD fluid inhibits leukocyte and macrophage function has led to the discontinuation of the practice of frequent initial lavages. Most physicians still carry out two or three quick in-and-out lavages, however. Some physicians use Ringer's lactate for these lavages (because this solution has a higher pH and lower osmolarity than PD fluid), and 200–500 U heparin/l is usually added.

11.1.2.2 Antimicrobial Therapy

Antibiotics, which can be added to the dialysate, are the mainstay of treatment. Several dosing regimens are used (see Table 11.5) [3], and the frequency of dosing

Table 11.5 Dosing of antimicrobials for peritonitis

Antimicrobials	Continuous dosing (mg/l)			Intermittent (once daily)
	Half-life CAPD (h)	Loading maintenance	All exchanges	
Aminoglycosides				
Gentamicin	32	8	4	0.6 mg/kg
Tobramycin	36	8	4	0.6 mg/kg
Amikacin	40	25	12	2 mg/kg
Netilmicin	18	8	4	0.6 mg/kg
Cephalosporins				
Cefazolin	30	500	125	15 mg/kg
Cefonicid	50	125	25	
Cefepime		500	125	1 g
Cephalothin		500	125	15 mg/kg
Cephradine		500	125	15 mg/kg
Ceftazidime	13	500	125	1 g
Cephalexin	9	500 po		250 qid po
Ceftizoxime		250	125	1 g
Cefamandole	8	500	250	500 d
Cefmenoxime	6	1,000	50	500 d
Cefoxitin	15	500	100	
Cefuroxime	15	500	200	200 od iv/po
Cefixime	15	200 po		200 d po
Cefoperazone	2.2	1,000	500	
Cefotaxime	2.4	1,000	250	1,000 d
Cefsulodin	11	500	25	250 d
Cerfizoxime	11	500	125	500 d
Ceftriaxone	12	500	250	500 d
Moxalactam	16	500	175	500 d
Penicillins				
Aziocillin		500	250	
Meziocillin		1,500 iv	250	1,500 bid
Piperacillin	2.4	2,000 iv	250	2,000 bid
Ticarcillin		1,000	125	1,000 bid
Ampicillin			125	
Oxacillin			125	
Nafcillin			125	
Amoxicillin		250–500	50	
Penicillin G		50,000 U	25,000 U	
Quinolones				
Ciprofloxacin	11	50	25	250 tid po
Fleroxacin	27	400 po		200 d po
Ofoxacin	25	200 po		100 d po
Others				
Vancomycin	92	1,000	25	15–30 mg/kg q5-7d
Teicoplanin	260	200	20	200 bid
Aztreonam	9.3	1,000	250	500
Clindamycin		150	150	
Erythromycin			25	250 qid po

(continued)

Table 11.5 (continued)

Antimicrobials	Continuous dosing (mg/l)			Intermittent (once daily)
	Half-life CAPD (h)	Loading maintenance	All exchanges	
Metronidazole	11	250 po/iv		250 tid po/iv
Minocycline			50 bid po	
Rifampin		300 po		300 d po
Combinations				
Ampicillin/sulbactam		1000	250	2 g q12h
Imipenem/cilastatin		500	200	1 g BID
Quinupristin/dalfopristin				25 mg/l in alternate bags
Antifungals				
Amphotericin		1.5	4	10–15 d iv
Flucytosine		1,500 po		500 d po
Fluconazole	72			75 mg 2d
Ketoconazole	2.4	200 po		100–400 od po
Miconazole		100		50–100

po orally, qid four times per day, d daily, od once per day, iv intravenous, bid twice per day, tid three times per day.

depends on the antibiotic. Smaller doses can be added to all dialysate bags or a larger single dose can be added to a single bag.

Generally, CAPD patients are infused with a loading dose of antibiotic in 1–2 l of dialysate. If patient has discomfort, the inflow volume is reduced to 1 l, otherwise 2 l if tolerated can be used with antibiotic in it. The inflow volume is reduced to about 1 l for the first few days (to reduce the patient's discomfort). The maintenance dose of antibiotic is continued in the dialysate using the patient's regular technique of CAPD or CCPD. This loading dose can be administered intravenously but the intraperitoneal route is preferred. Frequent exchanges (with shorter dwell time) are not indicated because this increases the cost of antimicrobials and fluid, and increases the loss of protein from the inflamed peritoneum.

Empiric antibiotic therapy: Before culture results are back, antibiotics should be initiated. The choice of antibiotic depends on the clinical condition of the patient and suspected organism (Gram staining may identify the organism). It is recommended that initially both Gram-positive and -negative organisms must be covered. Gram-positive organisms can be covered with either vancomycin or a first-generation cephalosporin (e.g., cefazolin). Gram-negative organisms can be covered by either third-generation cephalosporin or aminoglycoside. Initial concerns about vancomycin-resistant organisms have not been documented further; the many methicillin-resistant *Staphylococcus Aureus* (MRSA) organisms being cultured make it pragmatic to use vancomycin. Similarly, a short course of judicious use of aminoglycoside does not seem to reduce the residual glomerular filtration rate

(GFR), as was feared, thus, recent recommendations have changed. Still, aminoglycoside use should be limited and every caution should be used to avoid toxicity.

Continuous use of antibiotics uses the principle that the concentration of antibiotic in the dialysate is roughly equal to the desired therapeutic level in the plasma. An alternative approach (intermittent use) has also been used. Thus, vancomycin can be administered as 1–2 g/exchange, allowed to dwell for about 6 h, and repeated once every 4–5 days, however, the level should be monitored and the dose repeated once the concentration drops below 15 μg/ml. Similarly, aminoglycosides can be administered as 20 mg/l/day and their level should be monitored. Figures 11.1a and b show some of the steps used in the treatment of peritonitis and the recommendations of the ad hoc committee [3–5]. Usually, the treatment is continued for 7 days after the first negative culture or after the clearing of the effluent.

We generally use continuous antibiotic (added to each bag) for the first 24–48 h and after that switch to intermittent dosing. The intermittent dose should be added to the cycle with the long dwell (nighttime for CAPD and daytime for automated peritoneal dialysis [APD]).

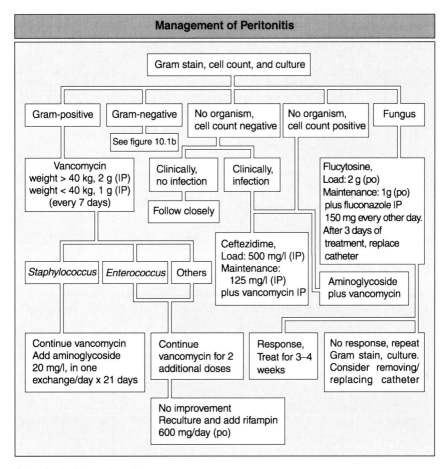

Fig. 11.1a IP intraperitoneal

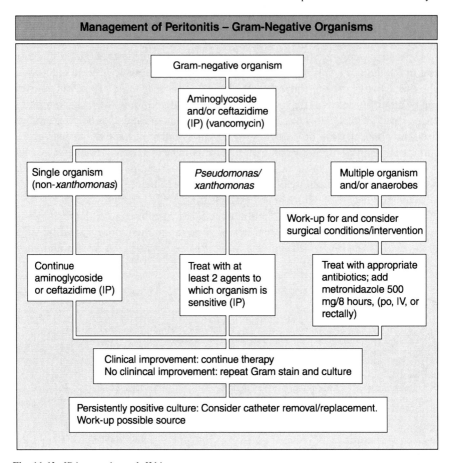

Fig. 11.1b IP intraperitoneal, IV intravenous

Coagulase-negative staphylococcus: This generally responds well to therapy. If the rate of MRSA is low in the population, first-generation cephalosporin (cefazolin at a 500 mg/l loading dose and a 125 mg/l continuous dose) can be used, but this should be used in all bags continuously. If MRSA is prevalent, vancomycin should be used (1 g/l, loading, repeated every 5–6 days). The usual length of treatment is 2 weeks.

Staphylococcus aureus: This usually is caused by touch contamination and is difficult to treat. Often, the catheter may need to be replaced. Vancomycin is usually used, however, the blood level should be maintained above 15 µg/ml. The treatment is longer, for 3 weeks with reculture to ensure eradication. An oral dose of rifampin (600 mg/day) added to another antibiotic for 1 week has been reported to be helpful. Rifampin should not be used alone. Linezolid, daptomycin, or quinupristin can be used to treat vancomycin-resistant organisms.

Pseudomonas aeruginosa: This infection usually requires a change of catheter. Oral ciprofloxacin with intraperitoneal ceftazidime can be used; alternatively, oral quinolone with tobramycin, piperacillin, or cefepime can be used.

For other Gram-negative organisms, select the antibiotic from the sensitivity profile.

11.1.2.3 Treatment of Fungal Peritonitis

Fungal peritonitis (and its successful treatment) is a challenging problem, seen usually in immunocompromised patients or in the setting of prolonged use of broad-spectrum antibacterial agents. Experience with oral and intraperitoneal antifungal agents such as the imidazoles has been good. One regimen uses intraperitoneal miconazole and oral fluconazole or ketoconazole for 3 to 4 days, after which, the old catheter is replaced and the antifungal therapy continued for another 2 weeks [4]. It has been suggested that if the symptoms improve and the culture becomes negative, the catheter may not have to be removed. In practice, however, replacement of the catheter is more successful in eradicating the infection.

11.2 Exit Site and Tunnel Infection (also see Chapter 9)

The most common organisms involved in exit site and tunnel infections are *S. aureus* or *pseudomonas*. Infection limited to the exit site and without purulent discharge can often be treated with local antibiotic alone. However, the presence of purulent discharge requires an oral antibiotic, the selection should be based on culture and sensitivity results. If the cuff is involved, purulent discharge when cuff is squeezed indicates more extensive treatment, often with the excision of the cuff. Usually a tunnel infection requires a change of catheter with a new tunnel under antibiotic cover.

11.3 Under-dialysis

Inadequate dialysis is a major problem and is an important cause of PD failure. When PD is initiated, patients often have residual renal function and combined PD and renal clearance provide adequate control of uremia. With time, residual renal function declines and peritoneal clearance alone may not be sufficient to provide adequate treatment. Thus, the loss of residual renal function is the most important contributor to inadequate dialysis. Other, less common causes of under-dialysis include poor compliance, improper technique, and loss of peritoneal membrane function. Anorexia, increasing fatigue, nausea and vomiting, insomnia, peripheral neuropathy, pericarditis, worsening nutritional status, and increasing requirement of erythropoietin (Epo) are common manifestations of under-dialysis. Initially, the blood urea nitrogen (BUN):creatinine ratio is low, suggesting lower protein intake, but with time there is loss of muscle mass and the creatinine concentration also declines. PD patients must be monitored regularly for nutritional status, dose of dialysis, and membrane function (see Chapter 10). At the first indication of inadequate dialysis, every attempt must be made to increase the dose. If this fails, the patient should be switched to some other form of renal replacement therapy (RRT).

11.4 Malnutrition

Protein malnutrition is prevalent in PD patients. The contributing causes include:

- Loss of amino acids and proteins in the peritoneal fluid
- Anorexia
- Increased calories from dextrose leading to reduced protein intake
- Increased intra-abdominal pressure, causing a feeling of fullness and decreased food intake
- Infections and concurrent medical conditions
- Under-dialysis

11.5 Membrane Failure

There are three types of membrane failure:

- Type I failure: In type I failures, high solute transport (see Chapter 10) causes failure of ultrafiltration (UF). This is due to quick absorption of glucose and the dissipation of the osmolarity of the fluid.
- Type II failure: In type II failures, sclerosing peritonitis and chronic ongoing inflammation cause decreased membrane permeability and surface area. This leads to decreased UF and solute transport.
- Type III failure: Type III failures are caused by excessive lymphatic absorption leading to a loss of net UF, with unchanged solute transport characteristics.

Type I membrane failure is the most common. Both types I and II can be characterized easily by peritoneal equilibration test (PET) results. Type III is a diagnosis of exclusion.

11.6 Cardiovascular Complications

Increased cardiovascular disease is seen in both hemodialysis (HD) and PD patients; left ventricular dysfunction, left ventricular hypertrophy (LVH), and cardiac arrhythmias all may occur. In new patients starting on CAPD, vasovagal reflex that

Table 11.6 Causes of Hemoperitoneum

Gynecologic	Gastrointestinal
Menstruation	Acute cholecystitis
Ovulation	Post-colonoscopy
Bleeding ovarian cysts	Intraperitoneal connective tissue pouch
Neoplastic	Catheter-induced splenic rupture
Renal cell carcinoma	Pancreatitis
Adenocarcinoma of colon	Miscellaneous
Polycystic kidney disease	Leakage from extraperitoneal hematoma
Hematologic	Tuberous sclerosis
Idiopathic thrombocytopenic purpura	IgA nephritis
Anticoagulant therapy	Mixed connective tissue disease
Peritoneal membrane disease	Extracorporeal shockwave lithotripsy
Peritoneal calcification	
Radiation-induced peritoneal fibrosis	
Sclerosing peritonitis	

Reproduced with permission from [6]

causes syncope has been described occasionally. The vasovagal reflex has been attributed to infusion of PD fluid into the abdominal cavity but it tends to disappear if the patient can be supported for a few weeks.

11.7 Intra-Abdominal Pressure

Increased intra-abdominal pressure due to extra peritoneal fluid can lead to the development of herniation of the abdominal viscera, back problems, and hemorrhoids. These complications are more commonly encountered in children and small patients.

11.8 Hemoperitoneum

Sometime, blood is seen in the peritoneal effluent. The most common cause of this in women of child-bearing age is menstruation, which is often associated with bleeding in the peritoneal cavity. Other causes are listed in Table 11.6 [6].

References

1. Goodman CE, Husserl FE. Etiology, prevention and treatment of back pain in patients undergoing continuous ambulatory peritoneal dialysis. *Perit Dial Bull* 1981, 1:119–122.
2. Anonymous. Catheter related factors and peritonitis risks in CAPD patients. *Am J Kidney Dis* 1992, 20(Suppl 2):48–54.

3. Gokal R. Peritoneal infections, hernias and related complications. In *Replacement of Renal Function by Dialysis*. 4th Edition. Edited by C Jacobs, CM Kjellstrand, KM Koch and JF Winchester. Dordrecht: Kluwer, 1996:657–688.
4. Johnson R, Ramsey PG, Gallagher N et al. Fungal peritoneal infections in patients on chronic peritoneal dialysis. *Am J Nephrol* 1985, 5:169–175.
5. Keane WF, Vas SI. Peritonitis. In *The Textbook of Peritoneal Dialysis*. Edited by R Gokal and KD Nolph. Dordrecht: Kluwer, 1994:473–503.
6. Bargman JM. Noninfectious complications of peritoneal dialysis. In *The Textbook of Peritoneal Dialysis*. Edited by R Gokal and KD Nolph. Dordrecht: Kluwer, 1994:555–591.

Chapter 12
Nutritional Issues

12.1 Protein Calorie and Nutritional Status of Dialysis Patients

Protein calorie malnutrition is common in dialysis patients, with as many as one third of patients manifesting mild or moderate malnutrition, and about one tenth manifesting severe malnutrition [1]. One study showed 45% of hemodialysis (HD) patients to have a protein intake of <1.0 g/kg/day [2], while another found this value to be <0.8 g/kg/day in 12% of patients [3]. The Morbidity in Maintenance Hemodialysis (MMHD) study [4] noted that the average caloric intake was 25–28 kcal/kg/day; substantially lower than the recommended intake of 35 kcal/kg/day. Patients who have protein–calorie malnutrition prior to the initiation of dialysis have a high risk of continuing in this malnourished state. In contrast, those who have good nutritional status prior to the initiation of dialysis maintain their healthy state. It is important to realize that the risk of malnutrition increases significantly with uremia and unless appropriate attention is directed promptly to this, malnutrition is inevitable. Anorexia and subtle manifestations of malnutrition develop when the glomerular filtration rate (GFR) declines to about 30 ml/min, progressing to significant malnutrition once the GFR falls to <10 ml/min. Because the influence of malnutrition on patient survival and well-being is so strong (see below), protein restriction during the predialysis phase has been controversial. In addition to protein and calorie malnutrition, other nutritional deficiencies are also encountered. These include deficiency of vitamins (including vitamins B and D), of trace elements (including iron, zinc, and selenium), and of other less understood substances such as carnitine. Table 12.1 lists the evidence for nutritional deficiencies in patients with uremia.

S. Ahmad, *Manual of Clinical Dialysis*, DOI 10.1007/978-0-387-09651-3_12,
© Springer Science+Business Media LLC 2009

Table 12.1 Nutritional indicators in dialysis patients

Parameter	Change from normal
Body weight (tissue, non-fluid)	Decreased
Growth and height (in children)	Decreased
Muscle mass	Decreased
Total body nitrogen	Decreased
Protein catabolism	Increased
Serum albumin	Decreased
Transferrin, prealbumin	Decreased
Essential amino acids	Decreased
Essential/non-essential amino acids	Decreased
Non-essential amino acids	Increased
Total body fluid weight	Increased
Free carnitine	Decreased
Acyl-carnitine	Increased
Acyl/free carnitine	Increased
Leptin	Increased

12.2 Significance of Nutritional Status

12.2.1 Hemodialysis

Several studies have shown that protein malnutrition in HD patients significantly increases the risk of death and hospitalization. In a report on the data from more than 13,000 patients, Lowrie and Lew [5] (see Fig. 12.1) showed serum albumin to be the most significant predictor of risk of mortality—with the odds ratio of death increasing several fold as serum albumin declined. An increase in mortality and morbidity (hospitalization) associated with evidence of protein malnutrition (as judged by low blood urea nitrogen [BUN] or protein catabolic rate [PCR]) has been reported [5,6]. Similarly, the Canadian Hemodialysis Morbidity Study found an increased risk of morbidity and mortality in the presence of low serum albumin [4], and both Owen et al. [7] and Collins et al. [8] found an increased risk of death with decreased serum albumin. In most of these studies, the risk increases when serum albumin is <3.0–$3.5\,g/dl$. Charra et al. [9] found that serum albumin $>42\,g/l$ was associated with a significantly better survival rate than serum albumin $<42\,g/l$ was, in their "very well dialyzed" patient group (see Fig. 12.2).

12.2.2 Peritoneal Dialysis

Data for chronic peritoneal dialysis (PD) patients is similar to that for HD patients. Longer survival is seen in those patients with higher serum albumin, PCR, and protein equivalent of nitrogen appearance rate (PNA), and the hospitalization rate is

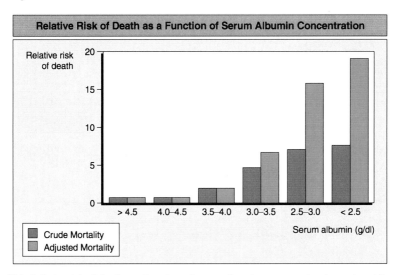

Fig. 12.1 Relative risk of death as a function of serum albumin concentration (reproduced from [5] with permission)

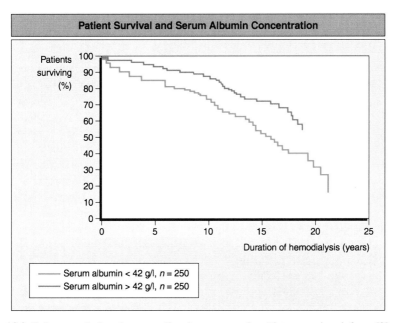

Fig. 12.2 Patient survival and serum albumin concentration (data reproduced from [9] with permission)

reported to be higher in patients with low serum albumin levels [10, 11]. A recent large study (from 10 centers and involving almost 700 patients) found serum albumin to be the strongest predictor of survival [12], with serum albumin of >3.5 g/dl associated with better outcome.

Thus there is strong emerging evidence that protein and nutritional status is a significant predictor of patient outcome in terms of both mortality and well-being. Therefore, dialysis patients with evidence of protein malnutrition (in the form of low serum albumin, urea concentration, urea appearance rate, or PCR) should be monitored and managed carefully. Similarly, patients with low serum cholesterol, creatinine, potassium, and phosphorus also have a poor prognosis [6], suggesting that their overall nutritional status influences outcome. This does not necessarily mean that increasing nutritional supplements and forced protein feeding will improve the outcome. A better understanding of the factor(s) causing the poor nutritional status and the correction of those factors, along with an improvement in nutritional intake, should be the goal.

12.3 Factors Causing Malnutrition

Multiple factors, including the underlying diseases, are responsible for a decline in nutritional status.

12.3.1 Uremia

Uremia is the cause of loss of appetite (particularly for protein-rich food) and is also associated with lower intestinal motility, gastritis, and ulceration, all of which can affect food intake and absorption. Bergstrom et al. [3] demonstrated a reduction in food intake in rats receiving an intraperitoneal infusion of uremic plasma ultrafiltrate. It was suggested that the anorexic fraction was in the 1–5 kd range—larger than the urea molecule and falling within the range to which the middle molecules (MMs) are assigned (see Chapter 6). Thus, it is possible that if dialysis aims to remove only small molecules such as urea, food intake problems will remain. Therefore, the appropriate therapy for protein malnutrition should be correction of uremia by adequate removal of toxin(s). As dialysis dose increases, the protein calorie nutrition improves [4]. It is possible, however, for a dose to be adequate in terms of urea clearance and yet have a relatively lower clearance of larger molecules (please note that, as discussed in Chapter 6, small molecule [SM] removal is influenced more by Qb and Qd, and MM removal by dialysis time). Provision of an adequate dialysis dose is especially critical in PD patients, in whom the protein and amino acids losses are significant and in whom overall uremic control is more dependent on the combination of dialysis and residual renal function.

12.3.2 Other Factors

Other important factors that influence the food intake in renal failure can be divided into three major categories:

1. Decreased intake:

   - Anorexia and decreased gastric emptying
   - Inappropriate dietary restrictions
   - Depression
   - Decreased intake on dialysis days
   - Inability to afford high-protein food
   - Altered taste
   - Medications affecting appetite such as pO_4 binders, iron,etc.
   - Underlying diseases such as diabetes, vasculitis, and psychosocial and emotional disturbances can lead to decreased food intake

2. Increased losses:

   - Loss of nutrients during dialysis—reused high-flux dialyzers have been reported to increase protein losses [13]. Protein losses during a bout of peritonitis in PD patients are quite large
   - Deficiency of water-soluble vitamins, which are easily dialyzed

3. Increased protein catabolism:

   - Inflammatory factors—production and release of cytokines and other inflammatory mediators can lead to increased protein catabolism
   - Metabolic disorders—disorders commonly associated with uremia, such as hyperparathyroidism, and increased glucagon, etc., can influence nutritional status
   - Metabolic acidosis—acidosis increases protein catabolism and may contribute to malnutrition
   - Intercurrent morbidities and hospitalization
   - Infections

12.4 Assessment of Nutritional Status

Several clinical and biochemical methods of assessing nutritional status are available and some of these are summarized below.

12.4.1 Dietary Intake

Dietary intake can be measured by using food diaries, dietary interviews, and urea/nitrogen appearance (UNA) rate to calculate dietary protein intake (DPI). Keeping a 2- to 7-day dietary diary under the direction of a trained renal dietician gives accurate information on nutrient and caloric intake. In stable patients who are not catabolic, there is a direct relationship between protein intake and total nitrogen output (DPI = PCR). The UNA rate is an accurate measure of the nitrogen output and can be calculated as the sum of all nitrogen lost during a fixed interval.

Thus, UNA/day equals the amount of urea in the dialysate and urine, plus the net increase in the total BUN in a day.
Or:

UNA $=$ (pre-BUN $-$ post-BUN) $\times$ (0.6 $\times$ weightpost) $+$ (weightpre $-$ weightpost) $\times$ pre-BUN $\times$ g/total time between two treatments, for hemodialysis,

where weightpost is the postdialysis body weight (in kilograms); weightpre is the next predialysis body weight (in kilograms); and pre-BUN and weightpre are measured immediately before the subsequent dialysis session.

PCR can be determined from UNA. Because most protein catabolism yields urea, the remainder of the protein loss in feces and sloughing of skin can be estimated (about 0.17 g/kg/day). Thus, the PCR for hemodialysis can be calculated by using the following formula:

PCR $(g/day) = 9.35 \times (G/BW) + 0.17,$

where G is the urea generation rate (in milligrams/minute) and BW is the patient's dry weight. Or:

PCR $(g/day) = 6.49 \times UNA + 0.294 \, V,$

where V is the volume of distribution of urea.

PCR can be normalized (nPCR) to the patient's weight, calculated from the urea space by using the following formula:

$$nPCR = 9.35 \times (G/V/0.58) + 0.17,$$

where G is the urea generation rate (in milligrams/minute) and V is the volume of distribution of urea.

Unlike HD patients, PD patients experience significant protein loss in the dialysate and have a significant urine output (often with large amount of protein). Therefore, the PCR is equal to the sum of urea appearance plus the total protein losses (in urine and peritoneal effluent). This measurement is the PNA, or, when normalized for body weight, the normalized PNA (nPNA). PNA is equal to PCR plus protein losses. In steady state, the PCR should be equal to DPI, however, studies in which the PCR is calculated from postdialysis and predialysis urea and urinary urea have not validated this relationship. This is most likely due to the variation in protein breakdown on dialysis and nondialysis days and error in calculation secondary to volume of distribution calculations. More importantly, the effect of PCR (DPI, UNA) on patient outcome has not been shown in studies. In the HEMO study controlling for creatinine and albumin, nPNA was not a predictor of outcome.

12.4.2 Anthropometry and Body Weights

Body weight, body mass index, and standard body weights can be used to estimate tissue mass. Lean body mass is a measurement of body weight without fat weight and has been used to determine the nutritional status in patients who do not have renal failure. In renal failure patients, increased water content makes this measurement difficult to use.

Fat-free and edema-free body weight can be calculated from creatinine production, the latter can be measured from urinary and dialytic losses in stable patients. The major nonrenal source of loss is from gut and can be calculated by:

Creatinine loss from gut = 0.036 × serum creatinine × body weight
Fat-free and edema-free body weight (in kilograms) = 0.029 × creatinine production (mg/day) +7.38

Skin fold thickness is a good indicator of total body fat. Measurement of the triceps skin fold thickness (TSFT) of the nondominant, non-vascular access arm is often used for this determination. However, in the presence of significant edema, this measurement is spuriously high. Mid-arm circumference correlates well with body muscle mass. Arm muscle area circumference (AMAC) can be calculated from the mid-arm circumference by using the following formula.

$$AMAC = (\text{mid-arm circumference [cm]}) - 0.314 \times TSFT \text{ (mm)}$$

12.4.3 Bioelectric Impedance Analysis

Bioelectric impedance analysis (BIA) measures fat mass, total body water, and non-fat tissues by measuring electrical resistance. Its usefulness in dialysis patients has not, as yet, been universally validated. However, low phase angle measurements have been reported to be associated with increased mortality. It is recommended that the measurements should be repeated within 2 h of the termination of hemodialysis.

12.4.4 Dual Energy X-Ray Absorptiometry

Dual energy x-ray absorptiometry (DEXA) measures the mineral density of bones using very little radiation and has been used to determine fat mass in various tissues. More work in dialysis patients is needed to validate this method.

12.4.5 Subjective Global Assessment

The subjective global assessment (SGA) is an inexpensive and easy method, and appears to yield reproducible results. It has been reported to correlate strongly with

Table 12.2 Biochemical markers for nutritional assessment

Biochemical Marker	Relationship	Remark
Serum albumin	Very strong predictor of outcome, minimum value 3.0–3.5/dl depending on measurement method	
Serum cholesterol	A value of <150 mg/dl is suggestive of malnutrition	
Serum transferrin	A value <2,000 mg/l may suggest malnutrition	Also influenced by infection and iron status
Serum prealbumin	In hemodialysis patients, prealbumin <0.3 g/l may suggest malnutrition	Acute decline in renal function may be associated with an increase in prealbumin, making the assessment difficult
Total body potassium	Correlates well with total body protein in nonrenal failure	This relationship is unclear in renal failure
3-methylhistidine	Reflects skeletal muscle protein degradation	

nutritional parameters, including serum albumin and BIA [14], and relates well to anthropometry and the PNA rate. In this technique, the medical history, physical examination, and protein calorie status are combined and a total score calculated. It has been modified for use in dialysis patients—four items are scored on a scale of 1–7 points [15]:

– Weight over the last 6 months (severe weight loss of >10% = 1–2; moderate weight loss of 5–10% = 3–4; and mild weight loss of <5% = 6–7)
– Anorexia
– Subcutaneous tissue (fat and muscle wasting)
– Muscle mass

12.4.6 Biochemical Assessment

Table 12.2 shows various biochemical markers that are used in the assessment of nutritional status.

12.5 Nutritional Requirements

Table 12.3 shows the recommended allowance for nutrients in dialysis patients [1]. Some of the major factors are discussed below.

Table 12.3 Recommended dietary nutrient intakes for patients undergoing maintenance hemodialysis or chronic peritoneal dialysis

Dietary nutrient	Maintenance hemodialysis[a]	Chronic peritoneal dialysis[a]
Protein	1.0–1.2 g/kg/day; >50% high biological value protein; 1.2/kg/day is prescribed unless the patient has normal protein status with intakes of 1.0–1.1 g protein/kg/day	1.2–1.5 g/kg/day; >50% high biological value protein; 1.2–1.3 protein/kg/day is generally prescribed for malnourished patients, up to 1.5 g/kg/day may be given
Energy (Kcal/day)	35%, unless the patient's relative body weight is >120% or the patient gains or is afraid of gaining unwanted weight;	35%, refers to dietary intake. Energy intake from peritoneal dialysate is in addition to these values;
Fat (percent of total energy intake)[b]	30–40	30–40
Polyunsaturated:saturated fatty acid ratio	1.0:1.0	1.0:1.0
Carbohydrate[c]	Remainder of non-protein, non-fat calories	
Total fiber intake (g/day)	20–25	20–25
Generals (range of intake)		
Sodium (mg/day)	1,000–1,500[d]	1,000–2,000[d]
Potassium (mEq/day)	40–70	40–70
Phosphorus (mg/kg/day)	8–17[e]	8–17[e]
Calcium (mg/day)	1,400–1,600[f]	800–1,000[f]
Magnesium (mg/day)	200–300	200–300
Iron (mg/day)	>/= 10–18	>10–18
Zinc (mg/day)	15	15
Water (ml/day)	Usually 750–1,500[d]	Usually 1,000–1,500[d]
Vitamins	**Diets to be supplemented with these quantities**	
Thiamin (mg/day)	1.5	1.5
Riboflavin (mg/day)	1.8	1.8
Pantothenic acid (mg/day)	5	5
Niacin (mg/day)	20	20
Pyridoxine HCl (mg/day)	10	10
Vitamin B_{12} (mg/day)	3	3
Vitamin C (mg/day)	60	60
Folic acid (mg/day)	1	1
Vitamin A	No addition	No addition
Vitamin D	See text	See text
Vitamin E (IU/day)	15	15
Vitamin K	None[g]	None[g]

Reproduced from [1] with permission

[a]When recommended intake is expressed per kilogram body weight, this refers to the standard weight as determined from National Health and Nutrition Examination Survey (NHANES) data or the adjusted body weight (ABW) for patients whose body weight differs by more than 15–20% from standard. ABW = standard weight + ([actual weight − standard weight] ×0.25)

[b]Refers to percent of total energy intake (diet plus dialysate)

[c]Should be primary complex carbohydrates

[d]Can be higher in continuous ambulatory peritoneal dialysis patients or in hemodialysis patients who have greater urinary losses

[e]Phosphate binders (aluminum carbonate or hydroxide, or calcium acetate, carbonate, or citrate) often are also used to maintain normal serum phosphorus levels

[f]Dietary intake usually must be supplemented to provide these levels

[g]Vitamin K supplements may be needed for patients who are not eating and who receive antibiotics

12.5.1 Protein

Protein intake of less than 1.0 g/kg/day is associated with a negative nitrogen balance, particularly on dialysis days [16]. HD patients should have a minimum daily protein intake of 1.2 g/kg, of which, 60% should be high biological value protein (e.g., poultry, fish, meat, and egg white). In catabolic states or in patients with losses of protein, the DPI should be increased above these values. There is a lack of data on the DPI in PD patients, but a minimum DPI of 1.3 g/kg/day has been suggested for continuous ambulatory PD (CAPD) patients. During the periods of peritonitis, when there is excess protein and amino acids loss, the intake should be increased.

12.5.2 Caloric Intake

The recommended caloric intake for average dialysis patient is about 35 kcal/kg/day. Usually the dialysis patient consumes less than the recommended calories and is in negative nitrogen balance. Every attempt should be made to provide sufficient calories to prevent protein catabolism.

12.5.3 Lipids

The common lipid abnormality in dialysis patient is hypertriglyceridemia with low high-density lipoprotein (HDL) cholesterol and an elevated low-density lipoprotein (LDL) fraction. Because of the increased prevalence of atherosclerosis, an abnormal lipid profile should not be ignored. The American Heart Association "step 1" diet requires that saturated fats should be limited to 20% and total calories from fat should not exceed 30%. The consumption of processed sugar and simple carbohydrate should also be limited, but the caloric requirements of 35 kcal/kg/day must be maintained (see above).

12.5.4 Fatty Acids, Lipids, and Carnitine

The prevalent lipid abnormalities and increased atherosclerosis that are observed in dialysis patients warrant special attention to this problem, but data on the use of L-carnitine to treat elevated triglycerides is controversial. A dose of >500 mg L − carnitine/treatment or per day is not usually associated with any improvement in triglyceride, and data with lower doses are limited and controversial. In summary, there is no clear evidence that L-carnitine reduces triglycerides or increases HDL cholesterol [17]. Limited data suggest that abnormalities in the fatty acid profiles (in some ways similar to essential fatty acid deficiency) of dialysis patients may commonly occur [18, 19]. Some improvements in fatty acid profile have been observed in a limited number of patients taking L-carnitine, but further investigation of this issue is necessary [20].

12.5.5 Vitamins and Trace Elements

Levels of water-soluble vitamins, folate, pyridoxine, and ascorbic acid have been reported to be low in dialysis patients. Their supplementation is common practice, with the recommended doses as follows: 1 mg folate/day, < 150 mg vitamin C/day, and 20 mg pyridoxine/day. Some authors have observed deficiencies at these levels and they recommend higher doses, but more work is needed to validate this finding. Increased levels of ascorbic acid have been associated with an increase in oxalate concentrations. Because dialysis patients generally have a higher oxalate load, larger doses of vitamin C should not be used.

Dialysis patients have a deficiency of active vitamin D (see Chapter 15) and an iron deficiency (on erythropoietin [Epo]) and need frequent supplementation (see Chapter 14). Zinc and selenium deficiencies have been reported and should be considered if a patient exhibits clinical manifestations. Data on thiamin, riboflavin, pantothenic acid, and biotin are limited.

Homocysteine is thought to directly damage vascular endothelium. Homocysteine levels are elevated in dialysis patients and higher levels have been found to increase the odds ratio for occurrence of vascular events [21]. Dialysis patients with vascular complications have been observed to have decreased blood concentrations of homocysteine after the administration of folate, and vitamins B_6 and B_{12}. These vitamins are co-factors in homocysteine metabolism. Folic acid at 5–15 mg/day has been shown to decrease homocysteine levels; however, its effect on vascular complications has not been elucidated [22]. Recently, 5 mg of 5-methyltetrahydrofolate administered orally has been reported to be more effective than folic acid in reducing homocysteine levels [23]. Supplementation of vitamin E is controversial (additional data are needed) and vitamin A should be avoided because it may cause toxicity in the dialysis population. Additional supplementation with vitamin K is not necessary.

The commercial preparation of vitamin and trace elements supplementation should be chosen carefully, and those containing vitamin A and/or higher dose of vitamin C should be avoided. Preparations containing large dosages of any vitamin or trace elements should not be used because this can lead to the accumulation of the vitamin and/or trace metal and subsequent toxicity.

Actual vs ideal (peer) body weight: Dialysis patients are usually malnourished and using their "unhealthy" lower weight would continue to provide inadequate nutrient and overestimate PNA (protein intake), thus, the malnourished state would be maintained, leading to poor outcome. It is recommended that for nutritional calculations the "peer" or desired weight should be used. The following example may clarify this point further.

A malnourished HD patient weighs 60 kg. He is 6 ft (72 in) tall. For his height and average build, his ideal weight should be 84 kg. Seventy-two grams of protein a day according to his current weight would be very appropriate at 1.2 g/kg, however, for the ideal weight of 84 kg, this amount would represent only 0.85 g/kg, or inadequate intake. Same calculations can be made for caloric and other intakes. For the same reasons, his nPNA would be overestimated because the volume of distribution of urea is calculated from lower malnourished weight. The use of correct weight for nutritional assessment is extremely important.

12.5.6 Additional Nutritional Support

Patients with clear evidence of malnutrition and those who are inadequately dialyzed may require additional nutritional support. First, an experienced nutritionist should interview the patient (and a close family member, if appropriate). If psychosocial elements or cultural factors are involved, these should be addressed appropriately. In the presence of inadequate dialysis, the dose of dialysis should be increased while nutritional counseling and help is continued. In a clearly malnourished patient who fails to increase food and calorie intake, additional oral supplements of protein and calories should be provided. Tube feeding, percutaneous gastric tube feeding, and parenteral feeding can be used in selected malnourished patients. Data on intradialytic parenteral nutrition (IDPN) is limited and controversial, and the additional costs that it entails should be considered prior to its use. Patients with low serum albumin levels have been reported to show improvement in mortality with IDPN, but in those patients with serum albumin >3.5 g/dl, there was an increase in mortality [24]. In another study, IDPN was associated with an improvement in nutritional profile but the mortality rate at 2 years was no different from that in the untreated group [25]. These results underscore the need for prospective, long-term, well-controlled clinical trials and the need to proceed cautiously in the use of IDPN.

12.5.7 Metabolic Acidosis

Renal failure is associated with metabolic acidosis, which improves with the initiation of dialysis. This is achieved by using a higher concentration of bicarbonate in the dialysate (usually 35–38 mEq/l). The blood bicarbonate concentrations are usually higher immediately after dialysis. The serum bicarbonate value prior to the HD session is, however, usually lower than normal. Patients' bicarbonate levels change from high–normal to subnormal (developing metabolic acidosis) at some point between the two dialysis treatments. Metabolic acidosis has been known to increase protein catabolism and cause a negative nitrogen balance. Correction of metabolic acidosis has been shown to improve protein metabolism in renal failure [26]. Improvement in muscle function in a group of HD patients has been reported with increased predialysis bicarbonate concentrations [27]. In patients with protein malnutrition, predialysis bicarbonate should be corrected to normal levels. This can be achieved by giving bicarbonate supplementation or by increasing dialysate bicarbonate concentration [28].

Intradialytic parenteral nutrition (IDPN): In a malnourished patient who is adequately dialyzed, sometimes IDPN is used for nutritional support. Its usefulness remains controversial, although one study observed decreased mortality with IDPN in those with serum albumin $<3.4\,g/dl$ [24]. The usual solution consists of 8.5% amino acid in 250 ml of 50% dextrose solution. The solution is slowly infused, usually in the venous drip chamber throughout the dialysis treatment. Rapid infusion may cause cramping of the access arm and may also precipitate hypoglycemia if the infusion is abruptly terminated. Hyperglycemia and hypoglycemia, hypertriglyceridemia, and infections are potential risks of the IDPN. Due to an increase in urea generation with IDPN, the Kt/V (K is the dialyzer urea clearance, t is the duration of dialysis, and V is the volume of distribution of urea) may decline (about 0.2) with IDPN.

Intraperitoneal amino acid: In PD patients who need nutritional support, 1.0% amino acid containing peritoneal dialysate can be used for long dwell (night dwell in CAPD and day dwell in automated peritoneal dialysis [APD]). The osmotic effect is similar to 2.5% dextrose solution. It is generally well tolerated, however, with more than one infusion, often anorexia, nausea and vomiting, and increased BUN is reported.

References

1. Fouque D, Kopple JD. Malnutrition and dialysis. In *Replacement of Renal Function by Dialysis. 4th Edition*. Edited by C Jacobs, CM Kjellstrand, KM Koch and JF Winchester. Dordrecht: Kluwer, 1996, pp. 1271–1290.
2. Jacob V, Le Carpentier JE, Salazano S et al. IGF-1, a marker of undernutrition in hemodialysis patients. *Am J Clin Nutr* 1990 52: 39–44.
3. Bergstrom J. Nutrition and adequacy of dialysis in hemodialysis patients. *Kidney Int Suppl* 1993, 41:S261–S267.
4. Eknoyan G, Beck GJ, Breyer JA et al. Design and preliminary results of the mortality and morbidity of hemodialysis (MMHD) pilot study [Abstract]. *J Am Soc Nephrol* 1994, 5:513.
5. Lowrie EG, Lew LN. Death risk in hemodialysis patients: the predictive value of commonly measured variables and an evaluation of death rate differences between facilities. *Am J Kidney Dis* 1990, 5:458–482.
6. Acchiardo SR, Moore LW, Latour PA. Malnutrition as the main factor in morbidity and mortality of hemodialysis patients. *Kidney Int* 1983, 24:199–203.
7. Owen WF, Lew NL, Liu Y et al. The urea reduction ratio and serum albumin concentration as predictors of mortality in patients undergoing hemodialysis. *N Engl J Med* 1993, 329:1001–1006.
8. Collins AJ, Ma JZ, Umen A et al. Urea index and other predictors of hemodialysis patient survival. *Am J Kidney Dis* 1994, 23: 272–282.
9. Charra B. Personal communication.
10. Teehan BP, Schleifer CR, Brown JM et al. Urea kinetic analysis and clinical outcome on CAPD. A five year longitudinal study. *Adv Perit Dial* 1990, 6:181–185.
11. Blake PG, Flowerdew G, Blake RM et al. Serum albumin in patients on continuous ambulatory peritoneal dialysis—predictors and correlations with outcomes. *J Am Soc Nephrol* 1993, 3:1501–1507.

12. Kashaviah P, Curchill DN, Thorpe K et al. Impact of nutrition on CAPD mortality. *J Am Soc Nephrol* 1994, 5:A494.

13. Donahue PR, Ahmad S. Dialyzer permeability alteration by reuse [Abstract]. *J Am Soc Nephrol* 1992, 3:363.

14. Enia G, Sicuso C, Alati G et al. Subjective global assessment of nutrition in dialysis patients. *Nephrol Dial Transplant* 1993, 8:1094–1098.

15. Churchill DN, Taylor DW, Keshaviah PR. Adequacy of dialysis and nutrition in continuous peritoneal dialysis: Association with clinical outcomes. *J Am Soc Nephrol* 1996, 7:198–203.

16. Borah MF, Schoenfeld PY, Gotch FA et al. Nitrogen balance during intermittent dialysis therapy of uremia. *Kidney Int* 1978, 14:491–500.

17. Ahmad S. Carnitine, kidney and renal dialysis. In *L-carnitine and its role in medicine. From function to therapy*. Edited by R Ferrari, S Dimauro and G Sherwoods. California: Academic Press, 1991, pp. 381–400.

18. Dasgupta A, Kenny MA, Ahmad S. Abnormal fatty acid profile in chronic hemodialysis patients: possible deficiency of essential fatty acids. *Clinical Physiol Biochem* 1990, 8:238–243.

19. Lacour B, Roullet JB, Drueke T. Les perturbations du metabolisme lipidique dans l'insuffisance renale chronique. *Nephrologie* 1983, 4:75–81.

20. Ahmad S, Dasgupta A, Kenny MA. Fatty acid abnormalities in hemodialysis patients: effect of L-carnitine administration. *Kidney Int Suppl* 1989, 36:S243–S246.

21. Dennis VW, Robinson K. Homocysteinemia and vascular disease in end stage renal disease. *Kidney Int Suppl* 1996, 57:S11–S17.

22. Yeun JY. The role of homocysteine in end stage renal disease. *Semin Dial* 1998, 11:95.

23. Bostom AG, Culleton B. Hyperhomocysteinemia in chronic renal disease: potential relevance to arteriosclerosis. *Semin Dial* 1999, 12:103–111.

24. Chertow GM, Ling J, Lew NL et al. The association of intradialytic parenteral nutrition administration with survival in hemodialysis patients. *Am J Kidney Dis* 1994, 24:912–920.

25. Capelli JP, Kushner H, Camiscioli TC et al. Effect of intradialytic parenteral nutrition on mortality rates in end-stage renal disease care. *Am J Kidney Dis* 1994, 23:808–816.

26. Williams AJ, Dittmer ID, McArley A et al. High bicarbonate dialysate in haemodialysis patients: effects on acidosis and nutritional status. *Nephrol Dial Transplant* 1997, 12:2633–2637.

27. Guest SS, Berenji MS, Kirsch CM et al. Functional consequences of correction of metabolic acidosis in hemodialysis patients. *J Am Soc Nephrol* 1997, 8:236A.

28. Ahmad S, Pagel M, Vizzo J et al. Effect of the normalization of acid-base balance on post dialysis plasma bicarbonate. *Trans Am Soc Artif Intern Organs* 1980, 26:318–321.

Chapter 13
Hypertension

It is of paramount importance that every attempt be made to control blood pressure (BP) in patients on dialysis because:

- Over 90% of patients initiating dialysis have elevated BP (defined as >140/90 mmHg)
- Cardiovascular disease is the most common cause of death in the dialysis population
- Hypertension increases the risk of left ventricular hypertrophy (LVH) and atherosclerosis
- Hypertension increases the risk of mortality significantly; conversely, control of hypertension increases survival

13.1 Prevalence

Based on casual predialysis BP measurement, 60–90% of dialysis patients have been reported to have hypertension (Fig. 13.1). Ambulatory BP measurements (24,48 h) have indicated that >70% of patients may have a diastolic BP >88 mmHg [1]. The prevalence increases considerably if patients taking antihypertensive medication are also counted as being hypertensive. The predialysis BP is better than the postdialysis BP as a measure of cardiac load and is the recommended measure to follow and control. Twenty-four-hour ambulatory BP seems to be more reflective of outcome measures such as LVH than casual clinic BP.

13.2 Control of Hypertension

The impact of BP control on renal and cardiovascular outcomes has been increasingly recognized. Thus, the 7th Joint National Committee on Prevention, Detection, Evaluation, and Treatment of High Blood Pressure (JNC7) recommends a target of

S. Ahmad, *Manual of Clinical Dialysis*, DOI 10.1007/978-0-387-09651-3_13,
© Springer Science+Business Media LLC 2009

<130/80mmHg in chronic kidney disease (CKD). Charra et al. [2, 3] reported that even in their largely normotensive patient group, those with lower BP values had significantly better survival rates (see Fig. 13.3). Several studies have emphasized the significance of BP control on patient outcome (Table 13.1).

However, in the presence of stiff arterial walls, the systolic BP target may be difficult to achieve and some think that a target of 140 mmHg in this group may be a reasonable value. However, the majority of dialysis patients are not reaching this target [4]. As seen in Fig. 13.2, only 30% of dialysis patients were at a target of 140/95 mmHg. The best survival data from Charra et al. suggests that lowering the

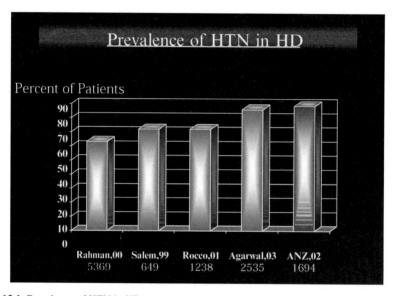

Fig. 13.1 Prevalence of HTN in HD

Table 13.1 BP has been found to be a strong predictor of outcome in dialysis patients in several studies, few of these are cited below:

> ➤ Charra (Tassin): Most Powerful Rx Related Predictor of Outcome was Pre-dialysis MAP
> •For Each 1 mm Hg Increase in MAP Risk of Death Increased by 3.9% (39% for each 10 mmHg)
> ➤ Foley: Each 10 mmHg Increase in MAP Risk of LVH Increased by 48%; & 5.4 g/m² LVMI
> ➤ Rocco: Odds Risk for Cardiomyopathy 2.64 in HTN Compared to NTN Pts.
> ➤ De Lima: In a group of 43 year old Pts. No Cardiac Hx, No Co-morbidities, HTN 2.2 Times More Likely to Die Than NTN Pts.

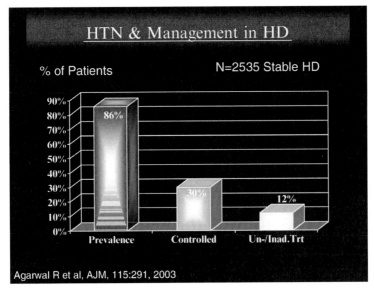

Fig. 13.2 Control of hypertension in dialysis patients [4]

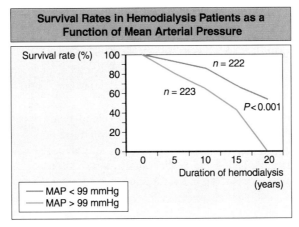

Fig. 13.3 *n*, number of patients, *MAP* mean arterial pressure (reproduced permission from [2] with permission)

BP without pharmacological agents should perhaps be the target of management of hypertension.

In a recent large international trial involving 19,000 patients with essential hypertension without renal failure, the optimum BP with lowest risk of cardiovascular event was found to be 138/82 mmHg [5]. Similar data for end-stage renal disease (ESRD) patients is not currently available. Klag et al. [6] looked at the risk of developing ESRD and found that with BP>127/82 mmHg, the relative risk of ESRD increased significantly.

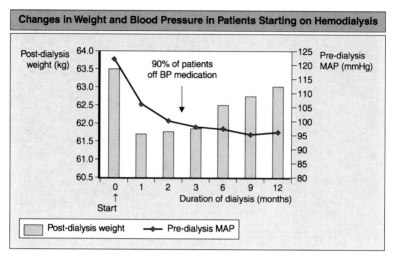

Fig. 13.4 *MAP* mean arterial pressure, *BP* blood pressure (reproduced from [2] with permission)

13.3 Significance of Hypertension Control

Cardiac dysfunction and atherosclerosis are common in dialysis patients and lead to increased morbidity and mortality [7]. From the results of Charra et al. [2, 3] (who demonstrated the best overall survival results in hemodialysis [HD] patients), several important observations can be made:

Hypertension is the most important risk factor for death in the dialysis population.

As discussed above, the risk of death increases significantly in patients with high normal BP, even in patients with well-controlled hypertension (see Fig. 13.3).

It is possible to control BP effectively with ultrafiltration (UF) and volume control and without antihypertensive medications in >95% of patients, with relatively slower and longer dialysis (Fig. 13.4). It is unclear whether the concurrent use of medications and volume control is associated with better control of hypertension than volume control alone. Survival data suggests that control of BP without medication is better and it makes sense that normal cardiac load with appropriate volume control should be better than carrying extra volume and using pharmacological agents to prevent any increase in BP. More work is needed to further clarify this important point.

13.4 Pathogenesis

An in-depth discussion of the factors involved in the pathogenesis of hypertension is beyond the scope of this chapter, but a summary is provided in Fig. 13.5 and some of the more important factors are discussed below.

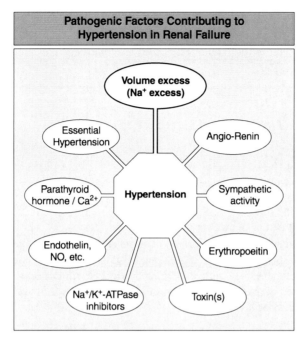

Fig. 13.5 There are a wide variety of pathogenic factors contributing to hypertension in renal failure. Volume excess (sodium excess) is the single most significant factor. *NO* nitric oxide

13.4.1 Sodium Excess

Sodium excess seems to be the most common cause of hypertension in dialysis patients. Plasma volume (PV), extracellular volume (ECV), and exchangeable sodium are all increased in patients with ESRD. The increase in ECV is larger in ESRD than in non-ESRD patients following a similar salt intake, and a reduction in sodium intake makes control of ECV and BP easier. Similarly, effective control of ECV and PV leads to a reduction (or even normalization) of BP. These observations emphasize the primary role of sodium in the pathogenesis of hypertension. There are several mechanisms by which sodium and ECV excess lead to hypertension:

Increased sodium increases ECV and PV, which leads to increased venous return, increased cardiac output, and reduced venous compliance.

Both an autoregulatory increase in total peripheral resistance (TPR) and a lack of a vasodilatory response to anemia cause elevation of BP. The factors responsible for these responses are:

(i) Increased media:lumen ratio of the arterial tree decreases the vasodilatory response
(ii) Increased circulatory endothelin increases the TPR
(iii) Decreased endothelium-derived vasodilators such as nitric oxide (NO) reduce the vasodilatory response

(iv) Increased sodium–potassium pump (Na^+/K^+–ATPase) inhibition, as a result of volume excess, leads to increased TPR
(v) Possible increased activity of Ca^{2+}–ATPase inhibitor leads to increased vascular tone and TPR

13.4.2 Other Factors

In patients with increased renin–angiotensin activity, BP control is easier following bilateral nephrectomy (seldom necessary since the availability angiotensin-converting enzyme [ACE] inhibitors, angiotensin II [AII] antagonists, and renin blockers). On the other hand, the use of erythropoietin (Epo) to treat anemia has been associated with a significant increase in hypertension.

Correction of anemia results in an increase in TPR and BP, and Epo also seems to have a direct vasoconstrictor effect. Elevated parathyroid hormone has been implicated in the pathogenesis of increased TPR and BP and arginine–vasopressin (AVP), which is elevated in dialysis patients and seems to be related directly to plasma osmolarity, may also be involved.

13.5 Treatment of Hypertension

The goal of hypertension therapy in dialysis patients is, as with nondialysis patients, to prevent end organ damage (e.g., atherosclerosis and LVH). Accelerated atherosclerosis [7] and LVH [8] are prevalent among dialysis patients. No long-term studies of the efficacy of various medications on regression of LVH have been carried out in the ESRD population, but good control of BP is associated with improvement in LVH [9]. In the non-ESRD population, the additional benefit of renin–angiotensin–aldosterone (RAA)-modifying agents beyond the BP control on cardiovascular outcome is well documented. Similar benefits of these agents in dialysis patients are also suspected; however, their use, unfortunately, in dialysis patients is limited. One reason for this may be related to the concern about hyperkalemia. As discussed above, the beneficial effects of normalization of the BP on survival is well documented [2,9]. The optimum level of BP has not been well defined, but data suggest that the target should be below 140/90 mmHg prior to dialysis [2].

13.5.1 Sodium and Volume Control

The most effective method to treat hypertension is by normalization of total body sodium and ECV. This is easier to achieve with continuous therapy, such as continuous ambulatory peritoneal dialysis (CAPD), or more frequent treatments, such as

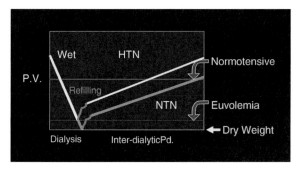

Fig. 13.6 Plasma volume and blood pressure with dialysis and during the inter-dialytic period (see text)

daily dialysis. For intermittent treatment, the first step of therapy is to limit dietary sodium intake (to about 2 g/day [88 mmol/day]), along with removal of excess fluid by UF to maintain appropriate dry weight. As seen in Fig. 13.6, if PV that is a part of ECV increases above the green line, hypertension will occur, however if PV remains under that line the BP will be normal. In this hypothetical example, during HD, the PV was decreased to the red line or euvolemia; however, because of the rate of UF being faster than movement of fluid from extravascular to the PV, some excess fluid will quickly move into the PV (equilibrate) after the treatment is stopped (shown by the blue line), and, during the interdialytic period with the continued salt and water intake the PV will continue to expand and after the green line passed, the BP will increase. Thus, to maintain normal BP during the entire interdialytic period, the PV (postdialysis weight or the dry weight) must be taken below the euvolemic level (orange line).

Dry weight: From above, the definition of dry weight could be "the weight at which the next predialysis BP is normal without any manifestation of fluid excess or depletion." It is interesting that when Thomson first described the dry weight in 1967, he wrote, "The reduction of BP to hypotensive levels during ultrafiltration represented the achievement of dry weight status." To this, the phrase "without antihypertensive medications" should be added.

To control BP, two requirements should be met, limit the interdialytic weight gain (IDWG) and dialyze long or frequently enough to remove all IDWG. The IDWG is determined by sodium intake because this leads to thirst and increased water intake. The emphasis thus should be to teach the patient to limit salt intake rather than continuous preaching of limiting water intake. As seen in Fig. 13.7, it is sodium not water intake that determines IDWG.

Patients need to recognize the salt content of foods and should learn how to avoid salt without sacrificing taste. Most patients who begin dialysis are hypertensive and are already receiving antihypertensive medications (including diuretics).

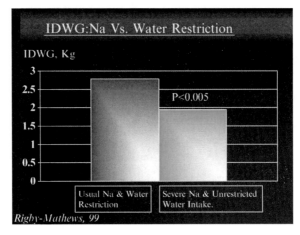

Fig. 13.7 IDWG:NA vs. water restriction

With advancing renal failure, diuretics are often less effective and higher dosages are required. The dose should not be increased to a toxic level.

13.5.2 Ultrafiltration

UF is the most important tool for normalizing fluid volume in dialysis patients and its judicious use can control hypertension in over 95% of patients [2]. Failure of UF to control ECV is usually the result of a rapid rate of UF. If UF is too rapid, PV depletion and its clinical sequelae (e.g., cramps, hypotension) occur, while extravascular volume and total ECV remain expanded. As soon as dialysis is stopped, an influx of fluid from the extravascular space causes the PV to expand and BP increases.

A typical patient spends 12 h of their 168 h/week (7%) on HD and the rest of the week (93%) free of HD. Consequently, patients with ECV expansion are hypertensive for the majority of time (in between dialyses). Slower UF with longer treatment is essential to the achievement of effective ECV control, maintenance of dry weight, and control of BP. Alternatively, more frequent dialysis also helps in controlling fluid weight and BP (Fig. 13.8).

A patient may need isolated or sequential UF and dialysis to achieve their true dry weight slowly. As dry weight is reached, a gradual tapering of the dose of antihypertensive medication will prevent the intradialytic hypotension that can limit UF. If short-acting medications are used, these can be withheld on dialysis days to make fluid removal easier, but the effects of long-acting medication last throughout dialysis even though the drug is not taken on the dialysis day. The patients described by Charra et al. [2] used longer and slower dialysis and UF. Buoncristiani et al. [9] used shorter but daily hemodialysis and achieved a good control of BP. These patients

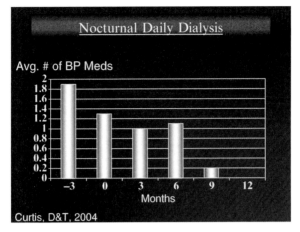

Fig. 13.8 Nocturnal daily dialysis

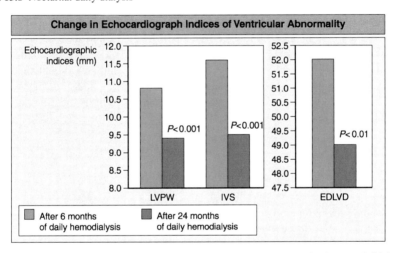

Fig. 13.9 *LVPW* left ventricular posterior wall thickness, *IVS* interventricular septal thickness, *EDLVD* end-diastolic left ventricular diameter (adapted from [9] with permission)

experienced significant improvements in left ventricular posterior wall thickness, interventricular septal thickness, and left ventricular diastolic diameter, with better control of BP (see Fig. 13.9). A practical scheme to control BP by achieving dry weight is shown in Table 13.2.

13.5.2.1 Hypertensive Response to Ultrafiltration

In some patients, BP increases (sometimes to a very high level) with UF. This paradoxical increase in BP has at times been mistaken for a sign of a patient being 'too dry," leading to discontinuation of UF. However, persistent UF and reduction of dry

Table 13.2 A suggested practical approach to a dialysis patient

On Antihypertensive	Hypertensive	Clinically ECV ↑
	UF	Slowly Decrease Postdialysis Weight

Hypotensive   Normotensive   Hypertensive

UF   Taper-off BP Meds.   UF

Hypertensive   Normotensive   Reduce & D/C
UF   *Dry Weight*   Beta-blocker
                                             Check K-Drop

Normotensive

Dry Weight

weight avoids this increase and leads eventually to better control of BP. This paradoxical increase in BP should not lead to discontinuation of UF. Every attempt must be made to further lower the dry weight. It is suggested (author's unpublished data) that discontinuation of beta-blockers may help to reduce dry weight further without cramps and/or increases in BP. Dialysis of antihypertensive medications has also been suggested as a possible contributor.

13.5.3 Pharmacological Agents

Various pharmacological agents are used in dialysis patients. First-line agents include calcium channel blockers (CCBs), ACE inhibitors, AII antagonists and beta-blockers. Second- and third-line agents include peripheral vasodilators, centrally acting sympatholytics, and alpha-blockers. Therapy should commence with a first-line agent, which, if BP is not controlled, should be supplemented with a second-line agent. If the maximum dose of the drug is ineffective, it should be discontinued and a new agent tried. Dose (and interval) should be adjusted for renal failure. Table 13.3 gives the kinetic details of commonly used antihypertensives [10].

13.5.3.1 Calcium Channel Blockers

CCBs block calcium channels in cardiac and smooth muscle cells and are perhaps the most commonly used antihypertensive drugs. The dihydropyridines (e.g., felodipine, amlodipine, nicardipine) have fewer cardiac and more peripheral effects and are thus better for control of hypertension. The major advantages of their use are listed below:

Table 13.3 Pharmacokinetics of the antihypertensives used in hemodialysis patients

	Elimination	T$_{1/2}$ (hrs) Normal/ ESRD	Plasma protein binding (%)	Dosing	Supplementation with dialysis	Miscellaneous
Diuretics						
Thiazides/ chlorthalidone	R			Avoid		
K$^+$ sparing						
Spironolactone	R			Avoid		K$^+$ sparing risk of hyperkalemia
Triamterene	H(R)			Avoid		Accumulate in uremia
Amiloride	R			Avoid		
Acetazolamide	R			Avoid		May potentiate acidosis
Loop agents						
Furosemide	R(H)			Useful in high doses	No	Ototoxicity and may augment aminoglycoside toxicity
Butetanide	R(H)			Useful in high doses	?	
Ethacrynic acid	H(R)			Avoid		
Beta-blockers						
Acebutolol	H(R)	8–9/7	10–20	25–50% of normal dose	No	Active metabolites accumulation
Atenolol	R	6–9/15–35	<5	25–50% after dialysis	Yes	Removed by dialysis
Labetalol	H	3–8/3–8	50	Unchanged	No	
Metoprolol	H	3–4/3–4	10	Unchanged	No	
Nadolol	R	14–17/36	20–30	50% of normal dose	Yes	Removed by dialysis
Pindolol	H(R)	3–4/3–4	40–55	Unchanged	No	
Propanolol	H	3.5–6/2.3	90–96	Unchanged	No	Active metabolites accumulation Interfere with bilirubin dosage
Sotalol	R	5–8/40–50	< 10	30% of normal dose	Yes	Class 3 antirrhythmic properties
Tertatolol	R	3/?	95	Unchanged	No	Active metabolites accumulation
Timolol	H	3–4/4	10	Unchanged	No	Inactive metabolites accumulation
Anti-adrenergic modulators						
Centrally acting						
Methyldopa	R (H)	1–8/3–16	< 20	Interval extension of dosage adjustment: 12-24 h	Yes	Active metabolites accumulation risk of prolonged hypotension
Clonidine	R	6–23/39–42	20–30	50% of normal dose	No	Risk of rebound hypertension
Peripherally acting						
Prazosin	H(R)	2–3/?	> 90	Unchanged	No	First dose effect. Renal failure decreases the amount of protein bound-chemical
Urapidil	H(R)	3/?	80	Unchanged	No	Inactive metabolites accumulation
ACE inhibitors						Anemia: Anaphylactoid reactions
Benazepril	R(H)	3/12	95	50% of normal dose	No	Non-renal clearance of Benazeprilate
Captopril	R	2–3/20–30	25–30	25–50% of normal dose	Yes	Active metabolites accumulation
Cilazapril	R(H)	3–60/>60	25–30	25% of normal dose	Yes	
Enalapril	R(H)	7/35	50–60	50% of normal dose	Yes	Patent drug accumulation
Fosinopril	R and H	4/20	> 95	Unchanged	No	ACE inhibitor undergoes 50% of hepatic elimination
Lisinopril	R	5–7/>5	10	25% of normal dose	Yes	
Perindopril	R(H)	5/27	20	25–50% of normal dose	Yes	
Quinapril	R(H)	2/17.5	97	25–50% of normal dose	No	
Ramipril	R(H)	5/15	60	50% of normal dose	?	

(continued)

Table 13.3 (continued)

		Elimination T$_{1/2}$ (hrs) Normal/ESRD	Plasma protein binding (%)	Dosing	Supplementation with dialysis	Miscellaneous
Trandolapril	R(H)	16–24/?	> 80	50% of normal dose	?	Trandolaprilat is further metabolized prior to excretion
Calcium-channel blockers						
Amlodipine	H	45/45	97	Unchanged	No	
Diltiazem	H	2–8/2–8	80–86	Unchanged	No	Risk of conduction disturbance
Felodipine	H	20–25/?	97	Unchanged	No	
Isradipine	H	2–8/8.5–14	95	Minimal dose available	?	
Lacidipine	H					
Nicardipine	H	1/1	95–98	Unchanged	No	
Nifedipine	H	4–5.5/4–5.5	92–98	Unchanged	No	
Nitrendipine	H	12/12	98	Unchanged	No	
Verapamil	H	3–7/2.4–4	85–95	50–75 Active metabolites accumulation	No	Negative inotropic effect
Vasodilators						
Diazoxide	R(H)	17–31/20–53	90	Unchanged	Yes	Smaller dose or slow infusion to avoid blood pressure decrease. Decrease of protein binding.
Hydralazine	H(NR)	7–4.5/7–16	87	Dosing interval prolonged 12–24 h	No	Induction of lupus-like syndrome Prolonged activity in slow acetylators
Minoxidil	H	2.8–4.2/3–4	0	Unchanged	Yes	Active metabolites accumulation
Nitroprusside	NR	< 10 mm/sam	0	Titrate by blood pressure	Yes	Accumulation of thiocyanate: need to monitor levels to keep <10 mg/dl. Thiocyanate is dialysable
AII antagonists	H					Risk of hyperkalemia
Losartan	H	4–5/4–5	> 98	Unchanged	No	
Candesartan	H	5–7/5–7	99	Unchanged	No	
Eprosartan	H	5–9/5–9	98	Unchanged	No	
Ibesartan	H	11–15/11–15	90	Unchanged	No	
Valsartan	H	6–9/6–9	95	Unchanged	No	
Tasosartan	H	0.9–6.6/0.9–6.6				
Telmisartan	H	13/13				

Adapted from [10] with permission
ESRD end-stage renal disease, *NR* nonrenal, *R* renal, *H* hepatic, *ACE* angiotensin-converting enzyme, *AII* angiotensin II

- Effective antihypertensives in dialysis patients
- Effect is more pronounced in the presence of fluid volume excess
- Are lipid neutral—no risk of increasing plasma lipid levels
- Effective in presence of hyperparathyroidism [11]
- May be protective against hyperkalemia [12]
- Metabolized by the liver (dose adjustment not required)
- Effective in improving arterial stiffness in the presence of calcification [13]
- 90% of the drug is protein bound and not dialyzed

In contrast, verapamil and diltiazem have more potent cardiac effects and less peripheral smooth muscle effects. For this reason, the non-dihydropyridines should not be used with beta-blockers because this combination can cause severe heart block.

The long-term effect of the CCBs on regression of LVH has not been defined but their use does have some disadvantages:

Constipation (a common problem in dialysis patients)

Facial flushing and headaches are common side effects but these tend to resolve if the medication is continued and patient is reassured

Development of ankle edema is common (not due to sodium retention)

Non-dihydropyridines are associated with heart block and congestive failure if used in conjunction with beta-blockers, or occasionally, if used alone

13.5.3.2 Angiotensin-Converting Enzyme Inhibitors

ACE inhibitors block the generation of AII and the degradation of the local vasodilator, bradykinin. Examples include enalapril, lisinopril, and fosinopril. They are effective in dialysis patients and have several potential benefits:

Dialysis patients have elevated peripheral renin activity; ACE levels are high and predialysis kallikrein levels are low. ACE inhibitors help to reduce the resultant increase in AII levels and increase kallikrein levels.

Elevated AII levels may contribute to LVH, and ACE inhibition will protect from this effect.

ACE inhibitors are the only drugs that have been shown to reduce LVH in dialysis patients [14] (others have not been evaluated).

Elevated AII levels have been implicated in excessive thirst and IDWG.

ACE inhibitors are lipid neutral and are only dialyzed partially. There are, however, certain potential disadvantages to the use of ACE inhibitors:

Severe anaphylactic reactions have been reported in patients who are taking ACE inhibitors and using dialyzers that contain acrylonitrile (AN)-6 membranes. Anaphylactic reactions have also been reported in patients using non-AN6 membranes. It is suggested that these reactions may be a result of the use of an inappropriately high dose.

Risk of hyperkalemia is high, and potassium levels need to be monitored carefully. These agents should not be used in patients at risk of hyperkalemia.

Side effects (usually minor) include cough, taste disturbances, skin rash, and (rarely) agranulocytosis (with captopril).

Because it is excreted by the kidney, drug dose adjustment is needed.

In summary, if used judiciously, ACE inhibitors have major advantages and may have some long-term benefits independent of BP control, such as resolution of LVH and reduction in thirst.

13.5.3.3 Angiotensin II Antagonists

Experience with AII antagonists (e.g., candesartan, losartan, valsartan) in dialysis patients is limited. Theoretically, they should have advantages similar to those of the ACE inhibitors, without some of the disadvantages. The risk of anaphylactic reaction is low, because AII antagonists have no effect on bradykinin degradation

Table 13.4 Comparison of ACE inhibitors and angiotensin II antagonists

	ACE inhibitors	Angiotensin II antagonists
Advantages		
Decreases angiotensin II level	Yes	No, decreases response to angiotensin II
Regression of LVH	Yes	Not studied in dialysis patients
		Reduces LVH in nondialysis patients
May reduce thirst	Maybe	Not studied
Lipid neutral	Yes	Yes
Disadvantages		
Anaphylactic reaction	Yes	Not reported
Cough as a side effect	Yes	No
Hyperkalemia	Yes	Not studied
Dose adjustment needed	Yes	No

ACE angiotensin-converting enzyme, *LVH* left ventricular hypertrophy

and there is no cough associated with their use. Experience in nondialysis patients shows that these drugs have effects on LVH regression that are similar to those of the ACE inhibitors. Current data on hyperkalemia in dialysis patients as a result of AII antagonist use is not available. AII antagonists are metabolized primarily by the liver and are only excreted partially by the kidney, thus, dose adjustment is not needed (see Tables 13.3 [10] and 13.4).

13.5.3.4 Beta-Blockers

These drugs lower BP by reducing cardiac output, and are used extensively in dialysis patients. Theoretical advantages to their use include their cardiac, anti-angina, and anti-arrhythmic effects. They also lower renin activity and have central adrenergic effects. However, these agents decrease HDL cholesterol, increase plasma potassium concentration, and block the symptoms of hypoglycemia in patients with diabetes. When these drugs are used, it may be difficult to lower dry weight to appropriate levels without causing intradialytic symptoms.

There are two types of beta-blockers: water-soluble (e.g., atenolol and nadolol) and lipid soluble (e.g., metoprolol). The half-life of water-soluble blockers is increased in renal failure and the dose needs to be adjusted accordingly. Water-soluble agents are also dialyzed well, and intradialytic hypertension and/or tachycardia may be a result of a drop in the blood levels. The lipid soluble beta-blockers are eliminated via the liver; however, some of their metabolites may be water-soluble and the dose may require adjustment (see Table 13.3).

13.5.3.5 Vasodilators

These drugs act directly on the arterial wall and decrease TPR and BP. Drugs in this class include hydralazine and minoxidil. These drugs are not commonly used because of their inability to reduce LVH and stimulation of reflex sympathetic activity. Minoxidil is a strong antihypertensive but carries the risk of pericardial effusion and congestive heart failure.

13.5.3.6 Central Sympatholytics

These drugs, examples of which include clonidine and methyldopa, act directly on alpha-adrenoreceptors in the brainstem and inhibit sympathetic outflow. They have several serious side effects and their use is limited. The greatest concern with these agents is the risk of rebound hypertension if a dose is missed. This is more common with the short-acting clonidine than with the long-acting methyldopa. Other side effects include dry mouth (clonidine), depression, postural hypotension, and sedation. Because these agents are excreted by the kidney, the dose needs to be adjusted.

13.5.3.7 Alpha-blockers

Prazosin blocks alpha-receptors but it is not a very potent antihypertensive and it causes postural hypotension. Labetalol, on the other hand, blocks both alpha- and beta-receptors and may be useful if both TPR and cardiac output are elevated.

13.6 Conclusions

After almost 40 years of treating ESRD with dialysis, hypertension remains prevalent and is responsible for a large number of deaths. Persistent and aggressive UF and a gradual withdrawal of antihypertensive therapy can be successful in controlling hypertension. In the words of Professor Scribner, "Adequate control of blood pressure now must become a part of the definition of adequate dialysis along with the adequate dose of dialysis and adequate intake of protein." The answer to Professor Friedman's question of whether hypertension in dialysis is "preventable or inevitable" [14] is that it is preventable and should be prevented.

References

1. Erturk S, Ertug AE, Ates K et al. Relationship of ambulatory blood pressure monitoring data to echocardiographic findings in haemodialysis patients. *Nephrol Dial Transplant* 1996, 11:2050–2054.
2. Charra B, Calemard E, Cuche M et al. Control of hypertension and prolonged survival on maintenance hemodialysis. *Nephrol* 1983, 33:96–102.
3. Charra B, Laurent G, Chazot C et al. Hemodialysis trends in time, 1989 to 1998, independent of dose and outcome. *Am J Kidney Dis* 1998, 32(Suppl 4):S63.

4. Agarwal R, Nissenson AR, Batlle D, et al. Prevalence, treatment, and control of hypertension in chronic hemodialysis patients in the United States. Am J Med 115(4):291–297, 2003.

5. Hansson L, Zanchetti A, Carruthers SG et al. Effects of intensive blood-pressure lowering and low-dose aspirin in patients with hypertension: principle results of the Hypertension Optimal Treatment (HOT) randomised trial. *Lancet* 1998, 351:1755–1762.

6. Klag MJ, Whelton PK, Randall BL et al. Blood pressure and end stage renal disease in men. *N Engl J Med* 1996, 334:13–18.

7. Haire HM, Sherrard DJ, Scardapne D et al. Smoking, hypertension and mortality in a maintenance dialysis population. *Cardiovasc Med* 1978, 3:1163–1166.

8. Harnet JD, Parfrey PS, Griffiths SM et al. Left ventricular hypertrophy in end-stage renal disease. *Nephron* 1988, 48:107–115.

9. Buonchristiani U, Fagugli RM, Pinciaroli MR et al. Reversal of left ventricular hypertrophy in uremic patients by treatment of daily hemodialysis (dhd). *Contrib Nephrol* 1996, 119:152–156.

10. London G, Marchais S, Guerin AP. Blood pressure control in chronic hemodialysis patients. In *Replacement of Renal Function by Dialysis, 4th Edition.* Edited by C Jacobs, CM Kjellstrand, KM Koch and JF Winchester. Dordrecht: Kluwer, 1996:966–990.

11. Raine AEG, Bedford L, Simpson AW et al. Hyperparathyroidism, platelet intracellular free calcium and hypertension in chronic renal failure. *Kidney Int* 1993, 43:700–705.

12. Solomon R, Dubey A. Diltiazem enhances potassium disposal in subjects with end stage renal disease. *Am J Kidney Dis* 1992, 19:420–422.

13. Marchais SJ, Boussac I, Guerin AP et al. Arteriosclerosis and antihypertensive response to calcium antagonists in end-stage renal failure. *J Cardiovasc Pharmacol* 1991, 18(Suppl 1):S74–S78.

14. Friedman EA (ed.). *Death on hemodialysis: preventable or inevitable?* Dordrecht: Kluwer; 1994.

Chapter 14
Anemia

The most common clinical problem associated with chronic renal failure is a reduction in the erythrocyte count, hemoglobin, and hematocrit (anemia). It was over 150 years ago that Bright first noted the presence of anemia in renal failure [1]. Once serum creatinine levels reach 3.0 mg/dl, most patients will experience a degree of anemia, and when dialysis is initiated, the majority of patients have anemia unless they are being treated with erythropoietin (Epo). Indeed, several of the clinical manifestations of uremia appear to be related in part to anemia. Correction of anemia usually improves tiredness, appetite, and quality of life.

14.1 Pathogenesis

The pathogenesis of anemia in renal failure is multifactorial but the most important contributing factor is a deficiency of Epo (see Fig. 14.1).

14.1.1 Erythropoietin

The normal kidney produces various hormones, one of which is Epo, a glycoprotein (molecular weight, 30.4 kd) that contains 165 amino acids and four carbohydrate chains. Renal peritubular capillary endothelial cells and interstitial fibroblasts appear to be the sites of renal Epo production. Epo binds to receptors on erythroid progenitor cells, allowing the cells to differentiate and proliferate, and leading to increased production of new red blood cells (RBCs). As renal parenchyma is lost, Epo production declines, causing a decrease in erythrogenesis by the marrow and leading to anemia.

Plasma levels of Epo vary widely (3–20 mU/ml in patients with uremia, and 3–26.3 mU/ml in non-uremic patients), but this variation may in part be due to the assay methods. Non-uremic anemic patients have higher levels of Epo than uremic

S. Ahmad, *Manual of Clinical Dialysis*, DOI 10.1007/978-0-387-09651-3_14,
© Springer Science+Business Media LLC 2009

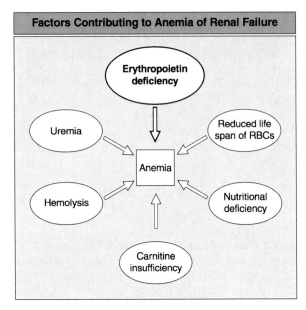

Fig. 14.1 Factors Contributing to Anemia of Renal Failure. *RBCs* red blood cells

patients with comparable levels of anemia. In general, uremic plasma appears to have lower Epo levels than normal plasma, although similar levels in both have also been reported [2]. The half-life of Epo depends on the route of administration: 4.5–0.9 h and 25–12 h following intravenous and subcutaneous administration, respectively [3].

About 90% of Epo is produced by the kidneys, with the liver (centrilobular hepatocytes) responsible for the other 10%. However, with renal failure, even a normal liver does not produce enough Epo to prevent a fall in hemoglobin levels. The number of circulating erythrocytes controls Epo production and secretion by a process of negative feedback, while positive feedback for stimulation of secretion is provided by hypoxia as a result of anemia.

14.1.2 Uremic Factors

Certain uremic factors in the plasma of dialysis patients are thought to inhibit production of erythrocytes (under the influence of Epo) and contribute to the anemia of renal failure. Clinical data show that hemodialysis (HD) patients dialyzed for longer durations have a higher hematocrit without Epo administration [4] than underdialyzed patients. Similarly, patients on continuous ambulatory PD (CAPD) have a higher hematocrit than those on HD. In the pre-Epo era, increasing dialysis in severely anemic patients resulted in an increase in hematocrit and reduced transfusion requirements in some patients. In vitro studies have shown the inhibitory effect of uremic plasma [5], and it has been suggested that certain molecule(s) that are larger than urea may inhibit the effect of Epo on progenitor cells. Thus, improving the efficiency of removal of uremic toxin(s) (by increasing the duration of dialysis treatment) should improve the erythrocyte count.

14.1.3 Other Factors

The life span of erythrocytes in uremia is shortened from 120 days to 60–90 days. Because Epo can treat renal anemia successfully, it has been suggested that this increased erythrocyte turnover plays a relatively minor role in the pathogenesis of anemia. No study of the effect of prolonging erythrocyte life span on anemia has been conducted, however. The reason for the shortened life span is unclear, but problems with the erythrocyte membrane may be responsible. Stabilization of this membrane by carnitine has been proposed as an explanation of increase in hematocrit with carnitine therapy (see below).

The increased loss of blood from the gastrointestinal tract and from dialysis procedures can lead to an iron deficiency anemia. With the use of Epo, the potential for iron deficiency has increased and iron supplementation is now a common practice. Other nutritional deficiencies can also contribute to anemia, but appear to be of minor importance.

14.2 Treatment of Anemia

14.2.1 Erythropoietin-Stimulating Agents (ESA) and Administration

In the USA, two types of Epo are currently available, epoetin alfa (Procrit, Epogen) and long-acting darbepoetin alfa (Aranesp). Another drug for continuous Epo receptor activator (CERA) has been approved by the US Food and Drug Administration (FDA) but at the time of writing is not available in the market. Because there are several different forms of the drug, the preferred term for this class of drugs is erythropoietin-stimulating agent (ESA). The three ESA are compared in Table 14.1

The anemia of renal failure should be treated with ESAs. It is important that other causes of anemia, particularly iron deficiency, are excluded before ESA therapy is initiated. In early clinical trials of intravenous 15–1500 mg Epo/kg (administered after each dialysis session), the dose–response relationship was shown clearly. Most patients responded to Epo doses in the range of 25–150 mg/kg/treatment, given intravenously.

Table 14.1 Comparison of Erythropoietin-stimulating agents

ESA agent	Description	Half life (h)	Dose frequency	Usual dose
Epoetin alfa	Recombinant erythropoietin	8.3	HD—three times/week	4,000–6,000 U/dose
			PD—once a week	8,000 U/dose
Darbepoetin alfa	Synthetic, with more carbohydrate; higher MW	24	HD—once a week	25 µg
			PD—2 weeks	60 µg
CERA		133	4 weeks	0.4–3 µg/kg

14.2.1.1 Route of Administration of Erythropoietin

Intravenous administration of Epo leads to a rapid peak plasma concentration followed by disappearance over the next 24–36 h (half-life, 4–9 h). Because the desired plasma levels are >50 mU/ml, the dose must be repeated at every dialysis session (three times a week). The subcutaneous route is becoming more popular because of the longer half-life (estimated to be 12–36 h) and better response following administration of Epo via this route. The major disadvantage of the subcutaneous route is the additional needle insertion, which some patients tolerate poorly. Intraperitoneal administration of Epo has been used with varying degrees of success. In this technique, the Epo must be administered to an empty peritoneal cavity and left in place for 12 h without exchanges of fluid. One group used 100 U Epo/kg intraperitoneally and obtained a serum concentration of Epo similar to that obtained with the subcutaneous route.

To continue stimulation of erythroid progenitor cells, the dose of Epo must be maintained. Complete cessation of the dose for even 1 week may suppress erythrocyte production (due to suppression of progenitor receptors) to a level below baseline and require a higher dose subsequently for a longer duration to increase the hematocrit. If the hematocrit increases beyond the target level (36% in USA), the intravenous Epo dose should be reduced by 25–50% (but the drug should be continued). With subcutaneous dosing, either the frequency or the magnitude of the dose can be reduced. If severe hypertension arises as a result of Epo administration, discontinuation is appropriate. It is preferable, however, to reduce the dose rather than discontinue it if the increase in the hematocrit is small or is not a direct result of Epo. Thus, in treating anemia, maintenance of the required dose at appropriate intervals is vital for a successful outcome. Current recommendations discourage raising the hematocrit above 39% or hemoglobin above 13 g/dl levels.

14.2.1.2 Lack of Response to Erythropoietin

There are three forms of Epo resistance:

Patients who fail to respond to Epo from the beginning of treatment

Table 14.2 Factors causing lack of response to erythropoietin

Factors	Management
Iron deficiency	Iron repletion
Active inflammation	Treat the cause, continue erythropoietin therapy
Severe hyperparathyroidism	Suppression or removal of the parathyroid
Osteitis fibrosa cystica	Treat hyperparathyroidism
Aluminum overload	Remove the source of aluminum and begin deferoxamine chelation
Carnitine insufficiency	Carnitine supplementation
Others: - Chronic blood loss and hemolysis - Nutritional deficiencies (folate, vitamin B_{12}, protein, trace elements, etc.) - Hemoglobinopathies - Angiotensin-converting enzyme inhibitors - Malignancies - Under-dialysis? (no direct data to support this)	

Patients who were responding normally and then become less responsive

Patients who require increasingly large dosages of Epo ($>150\,U/kg$) to maintain a hematocrit $>30\%$

There are several reasons for Epo resistance, iron deficiency being by far the most common (see Table 14.2). Once iron stores are replenished, hemoglobin increases with a lower dose of Epo. The presence of inflammation is the second most common cause of Epo resistance. This is associated with decreased serum iron, a decreased reticulocyte count, and increased ferritin levels. To avoid any delay in erythropoiesis when the inflammation subsides, the patient should continue to receive their usual dose of Epo. Severe hyperparathyroidism or osteitis fibrosa cystica can also increase the Epo dose requirement and, even with increased dose, the response is often poor. This usually improves soon after parathyroidectomy. Aluminum intoxication is also associated with resistance to Epo and presents with low mean corpuscular volume (MCV), normal iron status, and increased aluminum levels. Reducing the aluminum load (with deferoxamine [DFO]) usually restores the Epo response. Other causes of anemia (e.g., hemolytic anemia) can increase the Epo requirement, as can carnitine deficiency (see below) and inadequate dialysis.

14.2.1.3 Adverse Effects of Erythropoietin

Serious adverse effects of Epo are relatively rare, but increased blood pressure (BP) is the most common (see Table 14.3). Some increase in BP is seen in most patients but can be treated easily with adjustment of antihypertensive treatment (vasodilators such as calcium channel blockers [CCBs] are usually effective). The BP may,

Table 14.3 Adverse effects of erythropoietin

Adverse effect	Comment
Hypertension	Common, particularly with rapid increase in hematocrit
Seizures	Usually associated with increase in blood pressure
Vascular access clotting	Controversial, risk may be higher for PTFE graft and with higher dose. However, benefit outweighs any small potential risk
Hyperkalemia/hyperphosphatemia	Not supported by most of the studies
Increased heparin requirement	Controversial
Allergic reactions	Not reported

PTFE polytetrafluoroethane (Teflon)

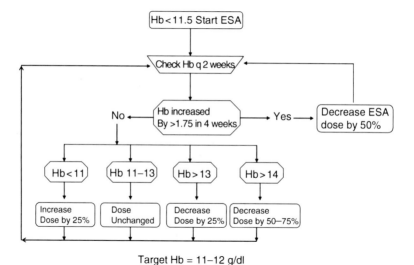

Target Hb = 11–12 g/dl

Fig. 14.2 Algorithm to treat anemia in dialysis patients

however, occasionally rise high enough to cause hypertensive encephalopathy. A small number of patients appear to be more sensitive to Epo and increased hematocrit, and, in these patients, BP control can become challenging. Increased total peripheral resistance (TPR) is the underlying hemodynamic abnormality causing an increase in BP [6]. Three studies have suggested that a higher hematocrit of >40% may be associated with increased mortality, and current guidelines recommend that the target hematocrit should be between 33% and 36% (hemoglobin, 11–12 g/dl). One possible scheme for adjusting dosage is shown in Fig. 14.2.

14.3 Iron Status

Prior to the availability of ESAs, dialysis patients were at risk of iron overload, mainly because of repeated blood transfusions. However, with the use of Epo, the risk of iron deficiency has become a real and common problem.

Despite the use of ESAs, only about half the dialysis patients in the USA have reached a hematocrit of 30% [7] (the current target for hematocrit is 33–36%). As discussed above, lack of iron is the most important contributing factor. The prevalence of iron deficiency is estimated at 43–90% of patients receiving Epo [7]. In the presence of normal marrow, erythropoiesis is dependent on Epo, iron, and folate. Diet and vitamin supplementation ensures that dialysis patients get enough folate, but the continued loss of blood (1 ml of red blood cells contains about 1 mg of iron) with dialysis and blood sampling, along with stimulation of erythrocyte production by Epo, easily leads to iron deficiency. Thus, continued supplementation with iron is needed.

14.3.1 Tests to Evaluate Iron Status

At present, none of the commonly used methods of assessing iron status in the dialysis patient are very sensitive or specific.

14.3.1.1 Ferritin

In the nondialysis population, serum ferritin is considered to be a reliable test of iron status ($<30\,\text{ng/ml}$ suggests iron deficiency). However, in patients with uremia, ongoing chronic inflammation or sequestration of iron in the bodily stores may mean that iron is not available for erythropoiesis (relative iron deficiency), even in the presence of a higher circulating ferritin level. A downward trend in serial serum ferritin measurements should alert the clinician to declining iron stores and corrective measures should be taken accordingly. In uremic patients receiving Epo, the lower acceptable limit for serum ferritin has been set at 100 ng/ml, but some propose that this should be 300 ng/ml and that a value below this should raise the possibility of iron deficiency.

14.3.1.2 Transferrin Saturation

In theory, the transferrin saturation represents the iron available for erythropoiesis. It is calculated by dividing serum iron by total iron-binding capacity (TIBC), which is essentially the circulating transferrin (TIBC [mg/dl] = transferrin [mg/dl] $\times$ 1.4), and this increases with iron deficiency.

$$\% \text{ Transferrin saturation} = \frac{\text{Serum iron}}{\text{TIBC}} \times 100$$

In non-uremic individuals, a transferrin saturation value of <16% is evidence of the presence of insufficient iron for erythropoiesis. In patients with uremia, a value of <20% has been shown to have a sensitivity of 88% and a specificity of 63% for the diagnosis of iron deficiency. It is important to note that exclusion of patients with hypoproteinemia increases the sensitivity and specificity to 100% and 80%, respectively.

A combination of serum ferritin and transferrin saturation is used widely to assess the iron status of a patient. A transferrin saturation of <20% and declining serum ferritin to <100 ng/ml are evidence of reduced iron availability and need for iron supplementation. The transferrin saturation should be targeted for 20–50% and ferritin 100–300 ng/ml to avoid an iron deficiency state.

14.3.1.3 Other Tests

Due to the problems with the diagnosis of iron deficiency, other methods of assessing iron status have been proposed, but most have limitations similar to those described above, are not widely available, or are expensive. One traditional test that seems promising is measurement of the percentage of hypochromic RBCs. Normally, <2.5% of erythrocytes are hypochromic, with a mean hemoglobin cell content of <28 g/dl. It is suggested that iron supplementation is necessary when >10% of cells are hypochromic [7].

14.3.2 Iron Supplementation

Total iron stores in women and men are, on average, 800 mg and 1,200 mg, respectively. If iron deficiency is absolute (as suggested by a ferritin level of <30 ng/ml and a percent saturation of <20%), intravenous iron (500 mg; single or divided dose) can be given; however, a lower saturation value (<20%) in combination with normal or elevated ferritin levels is often seen. This suggests that there is a deficiency of iron for erythropoiesis but either the iron stores are not yet depleted, the iron in the stores is not available for erythropoiesis, or inflammation is present. This relative deficiency needs to be treated with aggressive oral or intravenous iron supplementation. Serum ferritin of >500 ng/ml should be considered an indicator of increased iron stores, and iron supplementation should be discontinued.

Most dialysis patients using ESAs for anemia should receive 150–200 mg of oral elemental iron daily. However, it is difficult to maintain iron stores with oral doses and most patients require intravenous dosing. Several different oral formulations are available and there is no indication that any one is superior to the others. It is important to remember that enteric-coated formulations may release their iron beyond the duodenum or jejunum (which is where iron absorption occurs) and, as such, should not be used (the prescription should specify this).

Currently, three intravenous iron preparations are available, iron dextran, ferric gluconate, and iron sucrose. Iron dextran is associated with a higher risk of anaphylactic reaction; whereas, the latter two have lower risk and are more commonly used. Most patients require regular intravenous iron dosing, either by repleting the deficiency with 1,000 mg administered over 8–10 consecutive HD procedures in divided dosage, or by a weekly dose of 25–100 mg given every week to prevent iron deficiency. There are three concerns with intravenous therapy: anaphylaxis, potential for unusual microbiological infection, and oxidative stress. Anaphylaxis manifests as back pain, shortness of breath, flushing, hypotension, and shock. First-time use of iron should be checked with a smaller test dose. The iron can be used by microorganisms to grow, and there is concern about increased risk of infection with intravenous iron. However, this issue remains controversial. Oxidative stress caused by intravenous iron may potentiate accelerated atherosclerosis. Increased carotid artery wall thickness with intravenous iron has been reported.

Serum iron status must be monitored regularly and intravenous iron given as soon as a deficiency is indicated. Inadequate iron supplementation results in excessive use of Epo, and continued erythropoiesis under the effect of ESAs can lead to severe iron deficiency and its associated clinical sequelae. Some clinicians have used a regular weekly intravenous dose of 50–100 mg iron during dialysis to avoid persistent iron deficiency, but iron sensitivity must be tested for prior to the initiation of intravenous therapy. Oral iron should not be administered with any drugs that may bind with it and prevent absorption. In a preliminary report, iron added to the dialysate has been shown to be effective [8].

14.4 Carnitine

Most dialysis patients exhibit a deficiency of free carnitine and an excess of acylated carnitine. Studies with L-carnitine supplementation prior to the availability of Epo showed an increase in hematocrit in patients. After Epo became available, an increase in hematocrit occurred when carnitine was added to the treatment and studies have reported a decreased Epo requirement in patients being supplemented with L-carnitine (see Table 14.4) [[9]–[21]]. It is becoming increasingly clear that L-carnitine administration in dialysis patients is associated with an increase in hematocrit often permitting a decrease in Epo dose while maintaining the hematocrit at the same level.

Table 14.4 Hematocrit, erythropoietin, and carnitine

Criteria (with carnitine)	References
Studies showing an increase in hematocrit/hemoglobin	[9–18]
Studies showing a decrease in erythropoietin dose	[11, 14, 19]
Studies showing response in a subgroup only	
Hemoglobin increased only in those not on erythropoietin	[20]
Increased hematocrit and erythrocyte count in those older than 65 years	[19]

The exact relationship between carnitine, Epo, and hematocrit is unclear. One suggestion is that the erythrocyte membranes are unstable, resulting in a shortened life span and hemolysis. By stabilizing the erythrocyte membrane, carnitine decreases hemolysis and improves anemia [22].

Carnitine supplementation at 20 mg/kg intravenously after each dialysis or 1 g daily as a divided oral dose should be considered in patients with a poor response to Epo and in whom none of the factors discussed above are present. If plasma levels can be determined easily and reliably, a high ratio of acyl carnitine to free carnitine (>0.6) implies a need for supplementation. Treatment should be continued for at least 3–6 months because the response to carnitine takes weeks to develop. In one study, the hematocrit level declined 3 months after the discontinuation of carnitine [19].

14.5 Other Measures to Improve Hematocrit Response

Nutritional and vitamin deficiencies (e.g., folate and amino acids) may aggravate anemia and corrective measures should be taken. Before Epo became available, androgens were used to increase the hematocrit and they may now be used in an attempt to reduce the Epo dose and the associated expense. As discussed, under-dialysis can result in a worsening of anemia. Conversely, increased dialysis dose is associated with an improvement in anemia. In patients requiring a large dose of Epo and who are not deficient in iron or other nutrients, the dose of dialysis should be evaluated and the clearance of middle molecules (MMs) should be improved. This can be attempted by increasing the duration of dialysis and using dialyzers with good clearance.

Anemia has been one of the most challenging clinical problems in dialysis patients, but with the availability of Epo, the challenge has shifted to maintaining adequate iron stores, defining the route of administration of Epo, and deciding on the optimum hematocrit level for this chronically ill patient population.

References

1. Bright R. Cases and observations, illustrative of renal disease accompanied with the secretion of albuminous urine. *Guys Hosp Rep* 1836, 1:338.
2. Naets JP, Garcia JF, Toussaint C et al. Radioimmunoassay of erythropoietin in chronic uremia or anephric patients. *Scand J Haematol* 1986, 37:390–394.
3. London G, Marchais S, Guerin AP. Blood pressure control in chronic hemodialysis patients. In *Replacement of Renal Function by Dialysis, 4th Edition*. Edited by C Jacobs, CM Kjellstrand, KM Koch and JF Winchester. Dordrecht: Kluwer, 1996:966–990.
4. Charra B. Personal communication.
5. Wallner SF, Vautrin RM. Evidence that inhibition of erythropoiesis is important in the anemia of chronic renal failure. *J Lab Clin Med* 1981, 97:170.

6. Moritz JL, Jensen WM, Ahmad S. Prospective study in patients on low dose of recombinant erythropoietin (Epo): hematocrit (HCT), blood pressure and hemodynamic responses. *J Am Soc Nephrol* 1990, 1:403.
7. Fishbane S, Maesaka JK. Iron management in end-stage renal disease. *Am J Kidney Dis* 1997, 29:319.
8. Gupta A, Amin NB, Besars A et al. Dialysate iron therapy: infusion of ferric pyrophosphate via the dialysate in maintenance hemodialysis (HD) patients. *J Am Soc Nephrol* 1998, 9:251A.
9. Labonia WD. L-carnitine effects on anemia in hemodialyzed patients treated with erythropoietin. *Am J Kidney Dis* 1995, 26:757.
10. Labonia WD, Morelli OH, Gimenez MI et al. Effects of L-carnitine on sodium transport in erythrocytes from dialyzed uremic patients. *Kidney Int* 1987, 32:754–759.
11. Megri K, Trombert JC, Zannier A. Role of L-carnitine deficiency in persistent anemia of maintenance hemodialysis (MHD) patients treated by erythropoietin(EPO) [Abstract]. *Societe Francaise De Nephrologie Toulouse.* 1997; 153.
12. Barrillon D, Cassuto-Viguier E, Iordache A et al. Role of L-carnitine deficiency in persistent anemia of maintenance hemodialysis (MHD) patients treated by erythropoietin(EPO) [Abstract]. *Societe Francaise De Nephrologie Nantes.* 1992; 103.
13. Savica V, Bellinghieri G, Mallamace A. Value of carnitine in periodic hemodialysis. *Rass Med Interna* 1986, 7:293–307.
14. Nilsson-Ehle P, Cederblad G, Fagher B et al. Plasma lipoproteins, liver function and glucose metabolism in haemodialysis patients: lack of effect of L-carnitine supplementation. *Scand J Clin Lab Invest* 1985, 45:179–184.
15. Bellingheri G, Savica V, Mallamace A et al. Correlation between increased serum and tissue L-carnitine levels and improved muscle symptoms in hemodialyzed patients. *Am J Clin Nutr* 1983, 38:523–531.
16. Donatelli M, Terrizzi C, Zummo G et al. Effects of L-carnitine on chronic anemia and erythrocyte adenosine triphosphate concentration in hemodialyzed patients. *Curr Ther Res* 1987, 41:620–624.
17. Mioli V, Tarchini R, Boggi R. Use of D, L-, and L-carnitine in uraemic patients on intermittent haemodialysis. *Int J Clin Pharm Res* 1982, 2:143–148.
18. Trovato G, Ginardi V, Di Marco V et al. Long term l-carnitine treatment of chronic anemia of patients with end-stage renal failure. *Curr Ther Res* 1982, 31:1042.
19. Caruso U, Leone L, Cravotto E et al. Effects of l-carnitine on anemia in aged hemodialysis patients treated with recombinant human erythropoietin. *Dial Transplant* 1998, 27:498.
20. Thompson CH, Irish AB, Kemp GJ et al. The effect of propionyl L-carnitine on skeletal muscle metabolism in renal failure. *Clin Nephrol* 1997, 47:372–378.
21. Albertazzi A, Capelli P, Di-Paolo B et al. Endocrine-metabolic effects of l-carnitine in patients on regular dialysis treatment. *Proc Eur Dial Transplant Assoc* 1983, 19:302–307.
22. Matsumura M, Hatakeyama S, Koni I et al. Correlation between serum carnitine levels and erythrocyte osmotic fragility in hemodialysis patients. *Nephron* 1996, 72:574–578.

Chapter 15
Renal Osteodystrophy

All patients with advanced renal failure develop abnormal bone metabolism of varying degrees. The bone pathology is related to abnormalities in calcium, PO_4, vitamin D, and parathyroid hormone (PTH); metabolism of these are interrelated, and become abnormal with the loss of renal parenchyma. To understand the bone diseases in renal failure, a basic understanding of the pathophysiology of calcium and PO_4 metabolism, and homeostasis is necessary.

15.1 Pathophysiology of Renal Osteodystrophy

15.1.1 Vitamin D Metabolism

Two major factors lead to abnormality in vitamin D metabolism. First, cholecalciferol (vitamin D) from skin and diet is converted to 25-hydroxycholecalciferol (calcifediol) in the liver. This calcifediol is converted to the active form (calcitriol; 1,25-dihydroxycholecalciferol) in the kidney. Calcitriol synthesis decreases as renal parenchyma is lost through renal disease. Second, calcitriol synthesis is inhibited by high and stimulated by low serum PO_4 levels; PO_4 accumulation is common with the loss of glomerular filtration rate (GFR) and hyperphosphatemia inhibits active vitamin D synthesis by kidney and stimulates PTH secretion by the parathyroid gland (discussed below). The major actions of calcitriol are listed below:

- Increases the intestinal absorption of calcium and PO_4
- Works with PTH to increase mobilization of calcium and PO_4 from bone
- Decreases urinary excretion of calcium and PO_4
- Inhibits the synthesis and release of PTH through calcitriol receptors in parathyroid cells (vitamin D receptors [VDRs])

S. Ahmad, *Manual of Clinical Dialysis*, DOI 10.1007/978-0-387-09651-3_15,
© Springer Science+Business Media LLC 2009

The effect of calcitriol is therefore to increase serum calcium and PO_4 and make them available for mineralization of bone. In renal failure, there is a deficiency of calcitriol.

15.1.2 Phosphorus Retention

A declining GFR leads to retention of PO_4 and an increase in serum PO_4. This hyperphosphatemia has several effects

- Decreased ionized calcium (iCa, Ca^{2+}): The excess PO_4 may force the following reaction to the right, causing a small reduction in iCa:
  - **iCa + HPO$_4$ $\rightarrow$ CaHPO$_4$.** A decrease in iCa stimulates secretion of PTH, which decreases tubular reabsorption of the PO_4 and, in early stages of renal failure, reduces serum PO_4 and restores iCa levels.
  - **Increased PTH secretion:** PO_4 directly stimulates PTH secretion, directly and indirectly through its vitamin D lowering effect, the latter being a PTH synthesis inhibitor (see below).
  - **Decreased calcitriol production:** Hypophosphatemia stimulates the production of calcitriol by the renal parenchyma. Hyperphosphatemia inhibits calcitriol synthesis. Calcitriol is a potent inhibitor of PTH synthesis and release. Therefore, a decrease in calcitriol removes that inhibition leading to unchecked PTH increase.
  - **Direct effect of hyperphosphatemia:** PO_4 restriction in renal failure has been shown to reduce PTH levels without increasing iCa and calcitriol levels [2,3], suggesting a direct effect of PO_4 on PTH concentrations.
- Trade-off hypothesis: A hypothesis to explain the relationship between PO_4 retention and increase in PTH has been proposed (see Fig. 15.1) [4]. As PO_4 increases, there is a transient decline in iCa. This decline stimulates secretion of PTH, which normalizes the PO_4 by increasing renal clearance. Because of this, iCa levels are restored. This cycle is repeated with each decline in GFR and normal PO_4 and iCa levels are maintained at the expense of a continued increase in PTH. Eventually, the nephron loss is so severe that elevated PTH fails to decrease the PO_4 level and hyperphosphatemia and hypocalcemia persist. At this stage, elevated PTH may even increase PO_4 levels by mobilizing it with calcium from the bone.

15.1.3 Parathyroid Hormone

PTH is a single-chain polypeptide with 84 amino acids and a molecular weight of 9.5 kd. It is secreted in response to a decline in serum calcium levels (potent

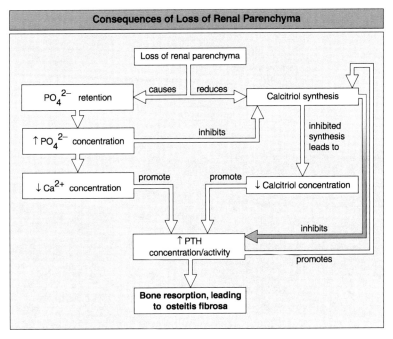

Fig. 15.1 *PTH* parathyroid hormone

stimulus) that stimulates calcium receptors, which in turn increase PTH synthesis and secretion. Changes in the beta-adrenergic system (less potent stimulus) also causes PTH increase. After secretion, PTH is fragmented into several inactive carboxy (C)-terminal fragments (7 kd; half-life, 25–60 min) and a small active amino (N)-terminal fragment in the liver and kidney. The major actions of PTH are listed below:

- Increases osteoclasts in bone, thus, increasing bone resorption (in the presence of calcitriol), and increases levels of calcium and PO_4.
- Increases renal synthesis of calcitriol, thus, increasing intestinal absorption of calcium and PO_4.
- Increases renal tubular reabsorption of calcium from the distal tubule and decreases tubular reabsorption of PO_4.
- Increases the number and action of osteoblasts thereby increasing bone formation.

As discussed earlier, there is increased secretion of PTH in renal failure, secondary to the factors listed in Table 15.1. This secondary hyperparathyroidism is common in dialysis patients and plays the central role in the pathogenesis of renal osteodystrophy (ROD).

Table 15.1 Causes of secondary hyperparathyroidism in renal failure

Phosphate retention
Hypocalcemia
Abnormal vitamin D metabolism and insufficient calcitriol
Resistance to the effect of parathyroid hormone (PTH) by the skeleton
Autonomous proliferation of parathyroid cells
Other factors

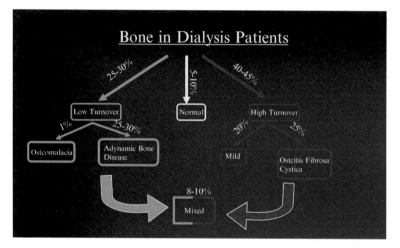

Fig. 15.2 Bone in dialysis patients

15.2 Histological Classification of Renal Osteodystrophy

Bone is a dynamic organ where continuous remodeling of the skeleton is carried out by osteoblasts and osteoclasts, both of which are regulated by hormones and local factors. Remodeling involves formation and resorption of bone. These processes are tightly coupled, and any alterations result in abnormal bone remodeling.

ROD is classified into three histological categories (Fig. 15.2):

– High-turnover disease: consequence of high PTH
– Low-turnover disease: Two subtypes—adynamic bone disease (ABD) and aluminum-related osteomalacia
– Mixed ROD [5]: Features of both high- and low-turnover disease

15.2.1 High-Turnover Bone Disease

High-turnover bone disease, caused by high PTH levels, is the most common type of bone disease, although the prevalence is declining. It is defined by increased rates of bone formation and bone resorption. The disease spectrum ranges from the mild disease in the presence of mild hyperparathyroidism, to osteitis fibrosa, where there is severe hyperparathyroidism. The more severe disease is usually seen with PTH > 500 pg/ml [6]. This is most common type of bone disease in dialysis patients, affecting 25–30% of patients. Bone biopsy shows marked activity, large numbers of osteoclasts surrounded by a large resorption cavity. Numerous osteoblasts are surrounded by a large osteoid mass without normal mineralization and endosteal fibrosis is commonly present. Tetracycline labeling shows two bands separated by a large new bone mass. Thus, there is a lot of bone formation and resorption activity with limited normal bone.

- Mild-to-moderate disease is asymptomatic
- Advanced disease:
  - Bone pain, joint pain, and pruritus
  - Bone tenderness, skin excoriation, palpable Ca deposits, and conjunctival redness
  - Elevated alkaline phosphatase levels (10 times), normal/low Ca or hypercalcemia not marked, elevated PO_4 (>6–7), PTH > 300 pg/ml (10–65), and elevated osteocalcin

15.2.2 Low-Turnover Bone Disease

Low-turnover disease is characterized by reduced numbers of osteoclasts and osteoblasts and low or absent bone activity. Osteomalacia is defined as decreased bone formation and excess unmineralized bone matrix (osteoid). At one time, osteomalacia secondary to aluminum toxicity was observed in dialysis patients, but with aggressive regular screening and avoidance of exposure to aluminum, the incidence has declined considerably, and currently, less than 1% of patients show it. However, low-turnover disease is increasing in certain patients such as those on peritoneal dialysis (PD). The ABD, which is seen in the absence of aluminum toxicity, has increased over the recent years. The lesion is similar to osteomalacia (but without excess osteoid accumulation), but the pathogenesis remains unclear. Patients with diabetes appear to be more prone to this problem. The serum PTH level is typically below 150 pg/ml [6, 7]. It is thought that one of the contributing factors may be oversuppression of PTH in susceptible patients.

- Low bone formation without osteoid accumulation (vs osteomalacia)
- Osteoblasts and osteoclasts decreased in number
- Low aluminum content

- Normal/low alkaline phosphatase and osteocalcin
- Associated with normal PTH, older age, diabetes mellitus (DM), steroid, fluoride, iron, acidosis, PD, hypothyroid, and Cushing's disease

15.2.3 Mixed (Uremic) Bone Disease

This disease is variable and has features of both high- and low-turnover disease, with one form predominant in some patients and the other form in the rest. The serum intact PTH (I-PTH) levels will depend on the predominant type of bone disease.

15.3 Clinical Manifestation of Renal Osteodystrophy

Patients with end-stage renal disease (ESRD) typically have more than one chronic illness and a heightened awareness is therefore crucial, especially when changes in the pattern of signs or symptoms are seen.

Pruritus and bone/joint pains are among the most common symptoms associated with ROD and Table 15.2 lists other symptoms. Factors such as secondary hyperparathyroidism, high calcium:PO_4 ratio, and the presence of beta-2-microglobulin are thought to be mediators of these symptoms. Secondary amyloidosis is a disease entity that develops in patients with ESRD who have been on dialysis for at least 5–10 years (incidence ranges from 30–100% [8]) be related to. Pathological changes occur as a result of amyloid deposition and are characterized by generalized arthralgias, bone cysts, periarthritis, joint effusion, lytic bone lesions, carpal tunnel syndrome (CTS), and, sometimes, tendon rupture and pathologic fractures. It has been suggested that the type of dialysis membrane used may be a factor and that the use of high-flux dialysis may reduce the risk for CTS [9]. There is evidence that the prevalence of the amyloidosis is declining over recent years, it may be because of more common use of high-flux dialysis and improved surveillance of bioincompatible factors in dialysis. Other causes of pathological fractures include aluminum bone disease and osteoporosis. There is now evidence that patients in this group have lower bone mineral density than age-matched controls, placing them at risk for fracture.

Table 15.2 Clinical manifestations of renal osteodystrophy

Dermatological	Musculoskeletal	Extraosseous calcifications
Pruritis	Generalized arthralgias	Periarthritis
Dry skin	Tendon rupture	Joint effusion
	Proximal myopathy or pathological fracture	Calciphylaxis
		Bone pain
	Carpal tunnel syndrome	

15.4 Metastatic Calcification

Deposition of calcium in soft tissue (non-osteal) such as in skin, eyes, around the joints, and in cardiac tissue and blood vessel walls are common and have serious implications. Calcium deposits in the cardiac tissue have been reported in the majority of dialysis patients on autopsy. Coronary artery calcifications are also common and may be responsible for the poor cardiovascular outcomes. The electron beam computed tomography (EBCT) technique has shown coronary artery calcification in the majority of dialysis patients. Elevated calcium, PO_4, and $Ca \times PO_4$ product are particularly responsible for the metastatic calcification. The practice of high-dose vitamin D therapy, large amounts of calcium-containing PO_4 binders, and high dialysate calcium bath may all be responsible for this condition.

Calciphylaxis or calci-uremic arteriolopathy (CUA), as the name suggests, is a form of soft tissue calcification involving the wall of the arterioles with endovascular fibrosis. The CUA is characterized by ischemic tissue necrosis, presenting as painful mottling or nodules, vascular calcification, and cutaneous ulceration [10]. The lesions may involve the toes, ankles, or fingers; these are called distal "acral" CUA. Often the lesions are more proximal, involving the thighs, trunk, and buttocks; these are called "proximal" CUA. As the disease progresses, the lesions progress into bleeding ulcers, and secondary infection, sepsis, and gangrene are common. Generally, the prognosis of the patient is very poor, especially with severe proximal involvement and with normal PTH. Small- and medium-sized arteries show histological signs of medial calcification and intimal hyperplasia. Although the pathogenesis of this syndrome remains unclear, it is probably multifactorial [11]. Severe hyperparathyroidism, high calcium $\times$ PO_4 product, and presence of uremia have been suggested as risk factors. Recently, morbid obesity and low serum albumin have been reported to be high risk factors, particularly for proximal calciphylaxis. The majority of recent patients have been reported to be morbidly obese patients with a body mass index (BMI) of > 35, most are women, and insulin-dependent diabetes may be an additional risk. The lesions often appear as a violaceous discoloration that progresses quickly to deep necrotic lesions and eschar formation. In some instances, lesions have responded to parathyroidectomy (PTX), but, in most cases, amputation is inevitable. Recent cases are different from those described earlier; the recent cases have close to normal PTH levels, $Ca \times PO_4$ product is greater than 60 mg/dl, and patients are obese and have proximal calciphylaxis with very poor prognosis. The optimal treatment is unclear, particularly when PTH is low or only mildly elevated. The following management plan is suggested:

- If PTH $> 600\,\mathrm{pg/ml}$, urgent PTX must be considered
- If PTH is not significantly elevated, use daily dialysis with low calcium dialysate (it is unclear at this point whether the use of citrate dialysate would have any added benefit)
- Stop all calcium intake, target PO_4 level to about 5.5 mg/dl or lower without calcium-containing binders
- Local wound management and antibiotic as needed

15.5 Laboratory Findings and Management of ROD

15.5.1 Laboratory Findings

15.5.1.1 Parathyroid Hormone

The accumulation of biologically inactive (i.e., mid-region and C-terminal) fragments of PTH may induce spuriously elevated levels of PTH in patients with ESRD. Assays to measure I-PTH by immunoradiometric assay (IRMA; Nichols Laboratories, San Juan Capistrano, CA) measures both active fragment (amino acids 1–84) and mostly inactive fragments of PTH. Optimal I-PTH levels by this method for uremic patients are considered to be between 100 and 300 pg/ml. Levels > 300 pg/ml and < 100 pg/ml are suggestive of high-turnover and low-turnover (adynamic) bone disease, respectively [2]. Recently, this issue has become more important with findings of elevated inactive fragments being inhibitors of PTH (amino acids 1–84) and downregulating the PTH receptors. Thus, higher levels of PTH may be necessary in uremia to produce normal effects of PTH. To address these, two more sensitive and specific assays have been developed to measure entire PTH but not fragments of amino acids. Nichols Laboratories has "Bio-intact PTH" and Scatibodies Laboratory (Santee, CA) "Cyclase Activating PTH (CAP)" or "bioactive PTH." The latter is more specific for only the active PTH. The target range for PTH in dialysis patients recommended by Kidney Dialysis Outcome Quality (KDOQ) are to maintain I-PTH between 150 and 300 pg/ml (16–32 pmol/L) or biointact PTH between 80 and 160 pg/ml (9–18 pmol/l).

15.5.1.2 Phosphorus

Phosphorus levels are elevated in the majority of patients with chronic renal failure and ESRD, with typical levels of 5.0–6.5 mg/dl. High levels reflect dietary noncompliance with PO_4 restriction and/or failure of PO_4 binders. Phosphorus itself is a poor predictor of the type of bone disease [12] and hyperphosphatemia may be associated with all three histological types of ROD. However, the hyperphosphatemia has more sinister effects, studies have shown it to be associated with a several-fold increase in relative risk of death. Thus, the reduction in PO_4 levels to a value below 6.0 mg/dl and $Ca \times PO_4$ product to a value below 60 mg/dl should be the target for all dialysis patients [13]. Factors causing hyperphosphatemia include:

Loss of GFR
Dietary PO_4 intake
Ineffective use of PO_4 binders
Frequency and efficacy of dialysis
Hyperparathyroidism—mobilizing PO_4 from bone
Use of vitamin D analogs, increasing PO_4 absorption from gut

The recommended serum PO_4 level is 3.5–5.5 mg/dl.

15.5.1.3 Calcium

Serum calcium levels are often low or normal in patients with ESRD. Hypocalcemia is seen typically in the presence of severe hyperphosphatemia. Recent use of a calcimimetic agent to treat hyperparathyroidism has become a common cause of lower calcium levels. Careful interpretation of low total calcium levels is important, especially in the presence of hypoalbuminemia (where ionized calcium levels may be normal or elevated). For calcium level corrected for serum albumin, the following formula can be used:

$$\text{Corrected Ca (mg/dl)} = \text{Total Ca, mg/dl} + (4.0\text{-albumin, g/dl})$$

Calcium is a poor predictor of the type of bone disease. Patients with low-turnover bone disease have higher serum calcium levels than those with high-turnover bone disease (even in the absence of aluminum toxicity), and the presence of hypercalcemia in this group warrants thorough investigation. The most common cause of hypercalcemia is excessive use of vitamin D analogs, but hypercalcemia in the presence of elevated levels of I-PTH may suggest autonomous hyperparathyroid tissue. Disease processes that are seen in the general population (e.g., malignancy, immobilization, or granulomatous disease) must also be considered (see Table 15.3).

The corrected Ca should be maintained in normal range (8.4 to 10.2 mg/dl); however, to reduce the risk of metastatic calcification, the preferred upper limit of Ca is 9.5 mg/dl.

15.5.1.4 Alkaline Phosphatase

Alkaline phosphatase levels reflect osteoid accumulation in the skeleton [14]. Elevated levels may be seen in high- and low-turnover disease but because a large number of patients have normal levels, serial measurements should be used to monitor disease progression. Bone alkaline phosphatase is a good marker for ABD, with low levels of this and low PTH ($< 150\,\text{pg/ml}$) having good specificity and positive predictive value. Further studies are needed to determine the cost-effectiveness of routine use of this test.

Table 15.3 Causes of hypercalcemia

Excessive use of vitamin D analogs
Severe hyperparathyroidism (autonomous parathyroid gland)
Aluminum bone disease
Malignancy
Granulomatous disease
Immobilization

15.5.1.5 Aluminum

Random aluminum levels above 50 g/l (measured by atomic absorption spectrophotometry) are suggestive of aluminum toxicity but levels below this do not exclude the presence of aluminum-related bone disease. In a recent study, 42% of the patients with biopsy-proven, aluminum-related bone disease had aluminum levels below 50 g/l, whereas 12% had levels below 20 g/l [15, 16]. Therefore, a cut-off level of 50 g/l for screening should be interpreted with caution, especially if the clinical suspicion is high. The presence of erythropoietin (Epo)-resistant anemia and PTH levels < 300 pg/l should raise the possibility of aluminum-related bone disease. Sources of aluminum include aluminum-containing PO_4 binders, the use of contaminated water during dialysis, and contamination of food during cooking with aluminum pots and pans.

The deferoxamine (DFO) test improves sensitivity and, in combination with PTH, < 200 pg/l is highly predictive of aluminum-related bone disease. Steps involved in the DFO challenge test are as follows:

1. Measure midweek serum aluminum level to establish baseline
2. Infuse 40 mg/kg DFO over 2 h during the last 2 h of dialysis

Collect a post-DFO serum sample at the start of the next dialysis (44 h later). A DFO test is deemed positive when the increment of aluminum levels is greater than 150 g/l. Close attention must be paid to the appearance of new or worsening of existing neurological symptoms. Once aluminum toxicity is confirmed, treatment with DFO at 5 mg/kg should be initiated (once weekly toward the end of the dialysis) and serum levels followed (once monthly during the 3-month course of therapy) [6]. If symptoms recur or the serum level is still elevated 1 month after completion of therapy, then therapy may be repeated.

15.5.1.6 Osteocalcin and Other Markers

Osteocalcin is a peptide that is secreted by osteoblasts and stored in bone matrix. It has been shown to correlate directly with bone formation in patients with ESRD. Studies suggest that osteocalcin may be useful in separating patients with high-turnover from those with low-turnover bone disease, but its high sensitivity and low specificity limit its usefulness as a marker for this differentiation. Moreover, the kidney excretes osteocalcin, and the products of osteocalcin degradation may be elevated in patients with ESRD, independent of bone formation.

Other biochemical markers of bone formation and resorption have been investigated, including procollagen type I C-terminal peptide (PICP) and cross-linked amino terminal telopeptide of type I collagen (NTx). Their clinical usefulness in determining the type of bone disease remains unclear.

15.5.1.7 Bone Biopsy

Bone biopsy is diagnostic tool for the diagnosis of ROD. However this being an invasive technique it is not commonly used. I-PTH measurement is currently the most useful noninvasive techniques for differentiating low- from high-turnover bone disease and has high positive predictive values when I-PTH levels are < 60 pg/ml and > 200 pg/ml, respectively [17, 18]. The indications for biopsy include pathological fracture (especially when PTH values are 60–200 pg/ml) and, in some instances, preceding PTX, to delineate the type of bone disease.

15.5.2 High Turnover Disease

15.5.2.1 Parathyroid Hormone Control

In vivo studies have shown that calcitriol suppresses PTH messenger RNA and therefore has a direct inhibitory effect on the parathyroid gland [19]. Furthermore, intravenous calcitriol suppresses PTH independent of calcium levels. The use of intermittent intravenous or daily oral calcitriol to control secondary hyperparathyroidism in patients with ESRD is a common practice. Both routes of administration produce good reductions in serum PTH levels but the incidence of hypercalcemia and hyperphosphatemia appears to be slightly greater with daily oral therapy (doses $> 0.5 \mu g$/day). Well-controlled comparisons of intermittent intravenous (5.25 µg divided in two doses) versus daily (0.75 µg/day) oral doses suggests very little difference [20] in effect between the two forms of administration. Two forms of vitamin D analogs are more commonly used because hypercalcemia and hyperphosphatemia are less common complications with these forms. Paricalcitol (19-Nor-1-alpha25-dihydroxyvitamin D [Zemplar]), and doxercalciferol (1a hydroxyvitamin D2 [Hectorol]) have mostly replaced the use of calcitriol to treat hyperparathyroidism. Oral forms of Zemplar and Hectorol are also available for patients who do not use injections [21]. The comparative dosages of intravenous vitamin D dosages three times a week are given in Table 15.4.

Calcimimetic agent: calcium-sensing receptors (CaSRs) are located on the surface of parathyroid cells, these receptors, on stimulation, reduce the production and release of PTH. Cinacalcet HCl is part of a new class of drugs that acts on the CaSRs and, by amplifying the response of these receptors to calcium, cinacalcet HCl effectively inhibits PTH. The PTH is inhibited and the resulting reduction in Ca and PO_4, in contrast to vitamin D treatment, is very desirable and may reduce the metastatic calcification over time. Long-term studies are underway to assess this possibility. The use of cinacalcet has made management of hyperparathyroidism much easier; however, the present cost of the medication remains the major barrier to its widespread use.

Table 15.4 Comparative dosages of intravenous vitamin D (three times a week)

PTH level (pg/ml)	Calcitriol, Calcijex (μg)	Paracalcitol, Zemplar (μg)	Doxercalciferol, Hectorol (μg)
> 400	1–2	2–6	4
Decreased by < 50% (level > 300)	increase by 1	increase by 1–2	increase by 2
Decreased by > 50%	Maintain	Maintain	Maintain
Level 150–300	Maintain	Maintain	Maintain
Level < 150	Stop	Stop	Stop

Table 15.5 Commonly used PO_4 binders

Agent	Examples	Usual dosages with food	Remarks
Calcium carbonate	TUMS, Oscal, Caltrate	No more than 1.5 g of elemental calcium per day	Least expensive, effective; Increase in Ca level limits its use
Calcium acetate	Phoslo, 667 mg/tablet	No more than 9 tablets a day	More expensive than $CaCO_3$; Similar risk of increasing Ca
Sevelamar	Renagel 400/800 mg	Often large dosages are needed	Less effective, no risk of increase Ca, associated with acidosis, expensive
Lanthanum carbonate	Forensol, 250, 500 mg	No more than 3,750 mg per day	More expensive, chewable
Magnesium carbonate	MagneBind 300 mg Mg and 250 $CaCO_3$	Dose limited by Mg levels	Dialysate Mg may need reduction

15.5.2.2 Phosphorus Control

Adequate control of serum phosphorus is essential for the prevention of soft tissue calcification and for management of secondary hyperparathyroidism. In healthy adults, the recommended dietary phosphorus intake is 1.0–1.8 g/d. In patients with ESRD, this value is approximately 800 mg/day. Further restriction of PO_4 may lead to protein deficiency unless the diet is supplemented with essential amino acids. Restriction of high-PO_4 foods (dairy products, most soft drinks) and the use of PO_4 binders with food (Table 15.5) will lower serum phosphorus levels in the majority of patients. Short-term studies have shown that calcium- and aluminum-free, nonabsorbable polymers (e.g., sevelemar hydrochloride) inhibit PO_4 absorption and these agents are now available [22]. Lanthanum carbonate is a very effective phosphate binder and is available as chewable tablets. No evidence of toxic accumulation has so far been reported with this agent. Prospective studies of long-term use of these agents are not available. Magnesium-containing antacids and iron salts have also been used as binders; however, the serum magnesium levels should be monitored closely to avoid hypermagnesemia. In cases in which this fails (due to the development of hypercalcemia or to noncompliance), aluminum-containing PO_4 binders over a short period may still play a role, as long as aluminum is closely monitored and they are not given with oral citrate. Table 15.5 gives the usual dosages of various commonly used binders:

Removal of phosphorus by dialysis is inefficient and cannot be solely relied on to control PO_4. However, developments such as hemodiafiltration and frequent dialysis seem to help in controlling PO_4 levels [23, 24]. Nicotinamide has been recently reported to decrease serum phosphate by interacting with phosphate absorption in the gut wall.

15.5.2.3 Calcium Supplementation

Calcium supplementation in patients with low serum calcium may be needed; however, with the common use of calcium-containing PO_4 binders and vitamin D, this often is not an issue. Manipulation of dialysate calcium may allow the use of higher doses of PO_4 binders.

15.5.2.4 Parathyroidectomy

In a minority of patients, surgical intervention remains the only treatment option. The indication for PTX is failure of maximal medical therapy that has resulted in one or more of the following:

- Severe hypercalcemia in the absence of other causes
- Pathological fractures
- Calciphylaxis with high PTH
- Severe symptomatic osteitis fibrosa

Three different surgical procedures can be performed: subtotal PTX (leaving the gland that is least hyperplastic), total PTX, and total PTX with autotransplantation. The short- and long-term complications vary according to the type of procedure. A careful and thorough intraoperative examination of the parathyroid glands should be performed to ensure the presence of four glands (8% of the population has more than four and up to 20% of the population has fewer than four parathyroid glands). There are reports of parathyromatosis complicating subtotal PTX and total PTX with autotransplantation [25]. It is recommended that most patients undergo subtotal PTX, with only those who are not candidates for future renal transplantation undergoing the total procedure [26]. Imaging studies such as technetium-99 m Sestamibi scintigraphy, ultrasound, or magnetic resonance imaging may have a role in the pre-operative localization of parathyroid glands.

15.6 Low-Turnover Disease

Low-turnover disease is becoming more challenging, particularly in high-risk patients (see above).

15.6.1 Aluminum Control

Reverse osmosis of the water used for proportioning dialysate has eliminated the problem of water being a source of aluminum. Oral citrate-containing agents should be avoided because citrate enhances the absorption of aluminum from the gut, and patients should not use aluminum kitchenware. There still appears to be a clinical role for aluminum-containing PO_4 binders. Their use should be limited and they should only be used in patients in whom calcium-containing binders have been shown to be inadequate or have resulted in hypercalcemia and other binders are not effective.

15.6.2 Low Parathyroid Hormone

The goal is to prevent oversuppression of PTH to a level below 150 pg/ml. This can be achieved by using appropriate dialysate calcium, higher calcium >2.5 mEq/l may cause the serum calcium to increase and suppress PTH. Low PO_4 levels inhibit PTH secretion and the PO_4 level should be kept in the normal range. A slight increase in PO_4 level to 4.5–5.5 mg/dl may stimulate PTH. Overuse of vitamin D and calcimimetics must be avoided and, when these are used, PTH should be closely monitored.

15.6.3 Other Therapies

Bisphosphonate can increase bone in osteoporosis but has not been properly tested in dialysis patients. These agents suppress osteoclasts and may further reduce bone turnover thus may not be appropriate to use in dialysis patients.

Teriparatide, a synthetic form of PTH (amino acids 1–34), increases density and may be of value in dialysis patients. More work is needed to establish its safety and efficacy.

15.6.4 Prevention

ROD continues to be a major challenge for the nephrologist, the patient, and other caretakers. Early restriction of PO_4 in the diet (even in the presence of normal serum phosphorus levels) may help to prevent the development of secondary hyperparathyroidism. The use of vitamin D early in the course of chronic renal failure is being proposed to prevent hyperparathyroidism but still remains controversial.

References

1. Rose BD, Rennke HG. Signs and symptoms of chronic renal failure. In *Renal Pathophysiology*. Edited by BD Rose and HG Rennke. Baltimore: Williams & Wilkins, 1994:276–300.
2. Lucas PA, Brown, RC Woodhead JS et al. 1,25-dihydroxycholecalciferol and parathyroid hormone in advanced renal failure: effects of simultaneous protein and phosphate restriction. *Clin Nephrol* 1986, 25:7–10.
3. Tessitore N, Venturi A, Adami S et al. Relationship between serum vitamin D metabolites and dietary intake of phosphate in patients with early renal failure. *Miner Electrolyte Metab* 1987, 13:38–44.
4. Bricker NS. On the pathogenesis of the uremic state. An exposition of the 'trade-off hypothesis'. *N Engl J Med* 1972, 286:1093–1099
5. Sherrard DJ, Hercz G, Pei Y et al. The spectrum of bone disease in end stage renal failure. An evolving disorder. *Kidney Int* 1993, 43:436–442.
6. Barata JD, D'Haese PC, Pires C et al. Low dose (5 mg/kg) desferrioxamine treatment in acutely intoxicated hemodialysis patients using two drug administration schedule. *Nephrol Dial Transplant* 1996, 11:125–132.
7. Couttenye MM, D'Haese PC, Van-Hool VO et al. Low serum alkaline phosphatase of bone origin: a good marker of adynamic bone disease in hemodialysis patients. *Nephrol Dial Transplant* 1996, 11:1065–1072.
8. Jadoul M, Garbar C, Noel H et al. Histological prevalence of beta-2-microglobulin amyloidosis in hemodialysis: A prospective post-mortem study. *Kidney Int* 1997, 51:1928–1932.
9. Koda Y, Nishi SI, Miyazaki S et al. Switch from conventional to high-flux membrane reduces the risk of carpal tunnel syndrome and mortality of hemodialysis patients. *Kidney Int* 1997, 52:1096–1101.
10. Gipstein RM, Coburn JW, Adams DA et al. Calciphylaxis in man. *Arch Intern Med* 1976, 136:1273–80.
11. Bleyer AJ, Choi M, Igwemezie B et al. A case control study of proximal calciphylaxis. *Am J Kidney Dis* 1998, 32:376–383.
12. Kates DM, Sherrard DJ, Andress DL. Evidence that serum phosphate is independently associated with chronic renal failure. *Am J Kidney Dis* 1997, 30:809–813.
13. Block GA, Hubert-Shearon TE, Levin NW et al. Association of serum phosphorus and calcium x phosphorus product with mortality risk in chronic hemodialysis patients: a national study. *Am J Kidney Dis* 1999, 31:607–617.
14. Couttenye MM, D'Haese PC, Van-Hool VO et al. Low serum alkaline phosphatase of bone origin: a good marker of adynamic bone disease in hemodialysis patients. *Nephrol Dial Transplant* 1996, 11:1065–1072.
15. Pei Y, Hercz G, Greenwood C et al. Non-invasive prediction of aluminum bone disease in hemodialysis patients. *Kidney Int* 1992, 41:1374–1382.
16. Antonsen JE, Hercz G, Pei Y et al. Random plasma aluminum is not useful in screening for aluminum bone disease. *J Am Soc Nephrol* 1997, 8:548A.

17. Malluche HH, Monier-Faugere MC. The role of bone biopsy in the management of patients with renal osteodystrophy. *J Am Soc Nephrol* 1994, 4:1631–1642.
18. Wang M, Hercz G, Sherrard DJ. Relationship between intact parathyroid hormone and bone histomorphometric parameters in dialysis patients without aluminum toxicity. *Am J Kidney Dis* 1995, 5:836–844.
19. Dusso AS, Brown AJ. Mechanism of vitamin D action and its regulation. *Am J Kidney Dis* 1998, 32(Suppl 2):S13–S24.
20. Quarles LD, Yohay DA, Carrol BA et al. Prospective trial of pulse oral versus intravenous calcitriol treatment of hyperparathyroidism in ESRD. *Kidney Int* 1994, 45:1710–21.
21. Martin KJ, Gonzalez EA, Gellens M et al. 19-Nor-1-alpha-25-dihydroxyvitamin D2 (Paricalcitriol) safely and effectively reduces the levels of intact parathyroid hormone in patients on hemodialysis. *J Am Soc Nephrol* 1998, 9:1427–1432.
22. Slatopolsky EA, Burke SK, Dillon MS. Renagal, a nonabsorbed calcium- and aluminum free phosphate binder, lowers serum phosphorus and parathyroid hormone. The Renagal Study Group. *Kidney Int* 1999, 55:299–307.
23. Mucsi I, Hercz G, Uldall R et al. Control of serum phosphate without any phosphate binders in patients treated with nocturnal hemodialysis. *Kidney Int* 1998, 53:1399–1404.
24. Ahmad S, Vizzo JE, Scribner BH. Reduction in aluminum load after one year of hemodiafiltration. *ASAIO Trans* 1986; 32:370–373.
25. Stehman-Breen C, Muihead N, Thorning D et al. Secondary hyperparathyroidism complicated by parathyromatosis. *Am J Kidney Dis* 1996, 28:502–507.
26. Alem AM, Sherrard DJ. Renal osteodystrophy. In *Principles and practice of dialysis, 2nd Edition*. Edited by WL Henrich. Baltimore: William & Wilkins, 1998, pp. 328–340.

Chapter 16
Atypical Dialysis Circumstances

Under certain unusual circumstances, specialized dialytic treatment is needed. Two examples are pregnancy and drug overdose.

16.1 Pregnancy

Pregnancy is uncommon in dialysis patients. The reported rate from different countries ranges from 0.3 to 3.4%, with the highest rate reported from Japan. The rate is at least twice as high in hemodialysis (HD) than peritoneal dialysis (PD) patients. The outcome of pregnancy was quite poor in the past but seems to be improving recently. The infant survival rate ranges from 25 to 57%. With more dialysis during the pregnancy, the infant survival seems to improve considerably. However, even surviving infants have high rates of complications: 85% premature births, >35% low birth weight (<1,500 g). Respiratory distress and congenital anomalies such as cerebral palsy and cortical atrophy are quite common.

16.1.1 Dialysis

In the past, HD was exclusively used in pregnant patients, however, for the last two decades, PD use has increased. Both therapies appear to be equally successful, the success rates being 44% versus 50% for HD and PD, respectively. PD being a continuous therapy avoids major perturbations in blood electrolytes and volume, however, during the later part of pregnancy, often the volume of fluid in the abdomen becomes more uncomfortable. The impact on the mother and fetus of high dextrose and lactate concentrations in the PD fluid have also not been fully explored.

S. Ahmad, *Manual of Clinical Dialysis*, DOI 10.1007/978-0-387-09651-3_16,
© Springer Science+Business Media LLC 2009

16.1.1.1 Hemodialysis

The success largely depends on overall dialysis delivered to the patients; infant survival improves with more dialysis. Greater than 20 h per week dialysis has better outcome than <20h per week. In one report, daily dialysis of 1.5–3.5 h was associated with 100% infant survival, however, a large number of patients were not on dialysis at the time of conception. Special consideration must be paid to the dialysis technique because increased dialysis and pregnancy together require major modifications in the dialysate bath and technique:

- Duration: >20h/week intermittent dialysis or daily dialysis with a minimum of 12 h/week; may need to increase the duration/freuency if the creatinine level is >3.5 mg/dL and the blood urea nitrogen (BUN) level is >45 mg/dL.
- Minimize large shifts in fluid by limiting the ultrafiltration (UF) rate (UFR)
- Patients are hypercoagulable, requiring heparin; if there is vaginal bleeding, reduce the heparin and consider citrate dialysate
- Dialysate modifications:

  - Increase the potassium concentration to 3–4 mEq/L to maintain predialysis plasma K in normal range
  - Decrease HCO_3 (25 mEq/L) to counter respiratory alkalosis
  - Usually, 2.5 mEq Ca/L is sufficient for calcium homeostasis
  - Increase Mg to 2.5–3.0 mEq/L maintain higher serum Mg levels
  - If serum PO_4 drops to low levels, it may have to be added in the dialysate bath. Two methods are:
    - Add 90 mmol sodium PO_4, injectable (Abbott Laboratories, Abbott Park, IL) in 3.7 L bicarbonate dialysate concentrate (3.66 mg/dl dialysate)
    - Add 54 (108 g) ml Phosphosoda (C.B. Fleet Company, Lynchurg, VA) laxative in 3.78 L of acid concentrate. If PO_4 level in blood increases above 5 mg/dL, the dialysate concentration should be reduced.

16.1.1.2 Peritoneal Dialysis

The over all dialysis has to be increased by at least 50%. This can be achieved by using automated peritoneal dialysis (APD) with multiple nightly cycler and several daytime exchanges. To improve comfort, often the inflow volume has to be decreased below 2 L and the exchange frequency increased to improve dialysis. No studies have compared minimum dialysate volume and fetal outcome. However, the serum concentrations of creatinine and BUN can be used as a guide. Peritonitis can be treated with cephalosporins or penicillins. If the outflow is bloody, the patient will need to be closely monitored to watch for spontaneous abortion or placental problems. Sometimes HD may need to be added to supplement PD in order to maintain creatinine and BUN concentrations in the desired ranges. If delivery is surgical, after surgery, the PD can be temporarily stopped or the inflow volume can be reduced with the peritoneum kept empty when the patient is not recumbent.

16.1.2 Associated Conditions

16.1.2.1 Hypertension

Over 75% pregnant dialysis patients have a blood pressure (BP) >140/90mmHg and/or require antihypertensive medications. More than 50% patients may have higher BP, in the 170/110 mmHg range. Accelerated hypertension requiring intensive care unit (ICU) admission is not uncommon, and at least one death with hypertension has been reported in this population. Thus, BP control is a challenging problem. The ideal method to control BP by fluid volume control, may be limited because of the risk of reducing uterine blood flow. It is customary to use fetal monitoring during dialysis and continue gentle UF to control extracellular volume (ECV). However, antihypertensive treatment may also be required. Angiotensin-converting enzyme inhibitors (ACEi) and angiotensin receptor blockers (ARBs) are contraindicated because of associated fetal anomalies. Alpha-methyl dopa and hydralazine have been used extensively in the past. In high cardiac output cases, beta-blockers and labetalol have also been used. Calcium channel blockers carry a risk of hypotension, and have not been generally used.

16.1.2.2 Anemia

Plasma expansion associated with pregnancy causes a significant decrease in hemoglobin/hematocrit in dialysis patients and the target hemoglobin for hemoglobin for pregnancy is 11 g/dl. This requires an increase in erythropoietin (Epo) dose by at least 50%. Complete blood count (CBC) and iron status need monitoring on regular weekly and monthly basis, respectively. The iron saturation should be maintained at >15% by the use of iron supplementation. If hemoglobin drops to 8 mg/dl, blood transfusion may be required.

16.1.2.3 Dietary Modifications

Phosphate and potassium restriction may have to be eased, this permits the higher protein intake that is recommended at 1.5 g/kg, and an additional 10 g of protein per day. Patients may not need phosphate binders, and the dry weight assessment must consider the normal fetal weight gain per week and, thus, it should be adjusted accordingly. Sodium should be restricted to reduce interdialytic weight gain to less than 2 L. The water-soluble vitamin dose needs to be increased fourfold.

16.2 Drug Removal in Overdose Situations

HD, PD, hemofiltration (HF), hemodiafiltration (HDF), and hemoperfusion are sometimes required in drug overdose and poisoning cases to remove the offending agent in order to protect the patient. These treatments should be used as an adjunct to other more effective and commonly used procedures, such as gastric lavage, activated charcoal, forced diuresis, and alkalinization of urine. First, the patient needs to be stabilized, the airway maintained, the temperature normalized, and the vital signs supported. After the diagnosis of the type of poisoning is made, the blood levels warrant reduction to safer level, if the agent is known to be removed by the extracorporeal method, and other usual methods have limited efficacy, the extracorporeal method must be used. Management of poisoning is beyond the scope of this book and other sources, such as the *Clinical Management of Poisoning and Drug Overdose* by Haddad et al. (1998) should be consulted [1].

16.2.1 Peritoneal Dialysis

PD is not as effective and is seldom useful in poisoning. However, if other therapies are not available and in small children, prolonged PD can be useful, particularly in cases of hypothermia, since it is effective in core warming.

16.2.2 Hemodialysis

For small, water-soluble molecules with limited protein binding, HD is very effective. Larger molecules such as vancomycin (1,500 Da) can be more effectively removed by high-flux dialyzers. Lipid-soluble drugs are not removed by hemodialysis. Sometimes prolonged dialysis or several sessions are needed to lower the blood level to less dangerous levels. Hemofiltration and hemodiafiltration can also be used if the volume of distribution is relatively small and a large volume procedure can be done. Most often HD with high-flux dialysis is quite effective.

16.2.3 Hemoperfusion

Use of a cartridge filled with adsorbant material such as activated charcoal or a resin is effective in removing highly protein-bound or lipid-soluble drugs. The cartridges are not always available and get saturated with time, if HD is equally effective, it is preferred over hemoperfusion. Sometimes a hemoperfusion cartridge has been used in series with a dialyzer to increase the efficacy. Several cartridges are available but activated charcoal (Table 16.1) has been most commonly used.

16.2.3.1 The Circuit

The hemoperfusion circuit is like a dialysis circuit with a cartridge in place of a dialyzer or in series with and prior to the dialyzer. The priming should follow the manufacturer's instructions for the device since they sometimes differ; for example, Gambro's instructions are to prime their charcoal column with dextrose to reduce the

Table 16.1 Hemoperfusion cartridges

Vendor	Device name	Adsorbant material/amount	Coated/material
Braun	Hemoresin	XAD-4/350 g	No
Asahi	Hemosorba	Charcoal/170 g	Yes/Ply-HEMA
Gambro	Adsorba	Charcoal/100, 300 g	Yes/cellulose acetate
Organon–Teknika	Hemopur 260	Charcoal/260 g	Yes/cellulose acetate
Clark	Biocomp, Syst.	Charcoal/50, 100, 250 g	Yes/heparin polymer
Smith & Nephew	Hemocol	Charcoal/100, 300 g	Yes/acrylic hydrogel

risk of hypoglycemia, but other manufacturers do not instruct to prime their device with dextrose. Often heparinized solution is used for priming to reduce clotting and thrombocytopenia. These devices require larger dose of heparin (5,000–10,000 U) to prevent clotting. The inlet for blood is kept down and the device is primed from below, the outlet for the blood is to be kept up.

The adsorbing surfaces of these devices get saturated and usually the device has a limited efficacy beyond 2–3 h, this period is usually enough to reduce the drug levels. Sometimes longer treatments are needed and the device should be changed every 3–4 h.

16.2.3.2 Complications

Thrombocytopenia, leucopenia, hypoglycemia, and some reduction in clotting factors are often noted with hemoperfusion. Usually these are transient and recovery occurs within the next 24–48 h. With high heparin dose and reduction in platelets and clotting factors, there is also a increased risk of bleeding.

16.2.4 Specific Examples

A few common instances are discussed below.

- Acetaminophen (151 Da) is a small water-soluble molecule, but oral activated charcoal and N-acetyl cysteine remain the most common management methods. Under unusual circumstances with very high levels, HD can be used.
- Salicylate (aspirin, 180 Da): The volume of distribution is only 0.15 L/kg and salicylate is 50% protein bound, however, if the serum level is >80 mg/dl (4.4 mmol/l) or if the blood level is >50 mg/dl and the patient has renal failure with unresponsive oliguria, HD should be considered and is quite effective.
- Barbiturates (232 Da): HD should be considered in cases with prolonged coma and high barbiturate levels. Since the drug has a low volume of distribution (0.5 L/kg) despite high protein binding, it is effectively removed by HD and hemoperfusion.

- Ethylene glycol and methanol: These are metabolized to produce formic and glycolic acids, respectively; glycolic acid is further metabolized to oxalate. All of these are toxic with significant noxious effects. These are quickly absorbed from the gut and have large volumes of distribution. HD is quite effective in removing alcohols as well as metabolites and should be considered, particularly in the presence of renal failure, severe metabolic acidosis, deteriorating vital signs, elevated levels, and worsening symptoms.
- Lithium (7 Da): HD is very effective in the removal of this small molecule with no protein binding. Due to a large volume of distribution (0.8 L/kg), long treatment is required and if rebound occurs, the HD should be repeated. Alternatively, continuous therapy such as hemodiafiltration can be used. HD should always be considered if the serum level is above 3.5 mmol/l or if renal failure is present and the level is > 2.5 mmol/l.

Reference

1. Haddad LM, Shannon MW, Winchester JF eds. Clinical management of poisoning and drug overdose, 3rd edition Philadelphia: WB Saunders, 1998.

Chapter 17
The Future

Several worrying trends are evolving in the field of end-stage renal disease (ESRD). A brief review of these is necessary to identify developments essential to the continued improvement in care provided to those suffering from ESRD.

17.1 Increasing Financial Pressure

The increasing incidence and prevalence of ESRD has led to a rapid and persistent growth of the ESRD population (currently estimated at well over one million worldwide). Because renal replacement therapies (RRTs) are supported, in the USA, largely by public funds, this is causing a heavy financial burden on national resources (the annual cost in the USA approaches $25 billion). This burden is likely to worsen unless some cost-reducing strategies are developed.

17.2 Changing Population

As life expectancies increase, the mean age of patients initiating dialysis is rising. Patients with diabetes, heart disease, and other comorbid conditions are living longer and are requiring RRT in increasing numbers. This population in particular will require "kinder and gentler" types of therapies.

17.3 Patient Outcome Measures

Patient mortality and morbidity rates have not improved substantially with time and there is some indication that they may even have declined in certain cases. The mortality rate in the USA continues to be worse than in Europe or Japan. In recent

S. Ahmad, *Manual of Clinical Dialysis*, DOI 10.1007/978-0-387-09651-3_17,
© Springer Science+Business Media LLC 2009

years, the 1-year mortality in the USA has improved but only by 2–3%. Several factors are responsible for this difference in patient outcome measures. Some of these are related to differences in the patient population, others to differences in treatment practices.

17.4 Limited Transplantation Options

The number of patients waiting for donated kidneys continues to rise, as does the waiting period. The existing method of kidney transplantation is unlikely to become the major form of RRT, and alternative methods must be developed because of the following:

- Limited number of organs available
- Surgical risk in an aging ESRD population, with comorbid conditions
- Side-effects of the currently used immunosuppressive agents

17.5 Low Rates of Rehabilitation

A large number of ESRD patients receiving maintenance dialysis have not returned to gainful employment. The consequences of this disappointing statistic adds to the financial burden to society. Major reasons for not returning to work are malaise, poor health (related to general condition), and lack of time (RRT and associated complications require frequent absences from work).

17.6 Ideal Renal Replacement Therapy

Keeping the above factors in mind, RRT should be:

- Flexible enough to meet the requirements of the individual patient in terms of schedule, type, and duration of treatment.
- Less expensive—so that the needs of the increasing patient population are fulfilled without a considerable increase in the financial burden to society. Unless overall costs are reduced, some form of rationing is inevitable.
- Associated with improved patient well-being, so that overall health and prognosis statistics improve.
- Associated with lower intradialytic and interdialytic complication rates. Transplantation rates can be increased by:
    - Increasing the acquisition of harvestable organs, by improved public education
    - Increasing the acceptance and use of "marginal" quality organs

– Use of xenotransplantation of organs
– Development of better antirejection therapies.

To reach the goals mentioned above, dialysis therapy has to change. Dialysis equipment should be made smaller, simpler, more automated, and more flexible. This will lead to increased self-care, longer (and perhaps slower) dialysis, and a better outcome. Increased self-care will reduce staffing costs (the largest cost component), thus, reducing the overall cost of care. Improved well-being and better health as a result of better treatment will reduce the costs related to treatment of the complications and sequelae of poor treatment (hospitalization). Improved health will also lead to increased rehabilitation and better financial return to society.

17.7 Simpler Machines and Daily Dialysis

Daily hemodialysis has long been considered to be better than intermittent three times a week dialysis [1], but an appropriate method of accessing blood on a daily basis is not currently available. This, along with the complexity of the current dialysis machines and costs associated with supplies, has limited the use of daily dialysis. Simpler hemodialysis machines that can enable more frequent dialysis and allow self-dialysis are currently under development by two groups. The machine by the Aksys group was geared for short, daily, home hemodialysis. Unfortunately this machine is not currently available. The machine by the Seattle group, Advanced Renal Technologies, is simple, automated, and can be used for center or home dialysis. It can be used daily or intermittently, using the single-needle or double-needle technique, and it has volumetric control features. Development and availability of these machines should provide additional flexibility in hemodialysis treatment and should result in cost benefits. Currently used NxStage machine at home is small portable and easy to use. However the machine uses lactate based dialysate at a very slow rate is only suitable for more frequent home treatments. The cost of the treatment is also quite high. However the machine has made it possible to send more patients home.

17.7.1 Diffusion vs Convection

The first step in decreasing the bulk of dialysis equipment is to move toward the widespread use of convective transport. Diffusive transport requires dialysate that increases bulk considerably and adds cost and complexity to the treatment. Generally, convection is better tolerated than diffusion.

17.8 Mechanical Artificial Kidney

The development of a wearable (and then an implantable) mechanical, artificial kidney (MAK) is a possibility. An artificial glomerulus is already available in the form of dialyzer/filter; the lack of a renal tubule equivalent, which would recover from the ultrafiltrate and reject the undesirable components is what is needed, has until now hindered the development of a MAK. The technology to develop a renal tubule does, however, exist, based on the concept of filtration. Using a second (more selective) filter, saline, which is the bulk of the needed solution, could be produced from the patient's own ultrafiltrate, thus generating the replacement fluid and reducing bulk of the system and the associated cost.

17.8.1 Implantable Mechanical, Artificial Kidney

Figure 17.1 shows the concept of an implantable mechanical kidney. The first filter (A) is connected to the circulatory access and filters plasma water that is then

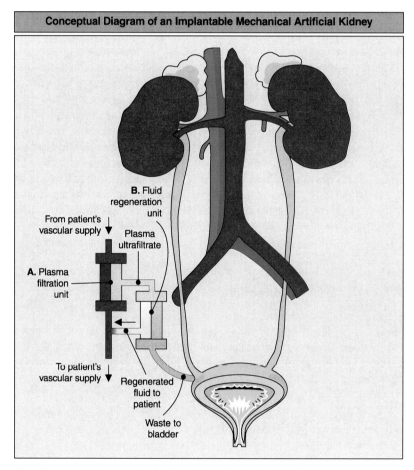

Fig. 17.1 Conceptual diagram of an implantable mechanical artificial kidney

channeled to filter B. This second filter (mechanical/biological reprocessor) allows the passage of sodium, other electrolytes, and water but retains urea and anything larger. Rejected "waste" from this unit is directed to the urinary bladder where it is periodically eliminated. The "good" portion of the ultrafiltrate can be returned to the postfilter (venous) portion of the vascular access.

As discussed above, the technology needed to develop an implantable MAK is available but lack of appropriate vascular access could pose problems. Connection of the device to the bladder should not be a major problem but connection to the vascular tree could be a major challenge. With the development of new ideas and with the use of currently available resources, an ideal access can, however, be developed. In the meantime, improvement of the existing and/or development of new dialysis equipment should continue, to address the problems previously discussed.

Recycling of uremic toxins: Another exciting development would be to use genetically altered bacteria to recycle uremic waste including urea and others, phosphate, etc., to produce amino acids and other nutrients in the gut. Some promising work is proceeding in this arena. A capsule containing these bacteria and adsorbants to adsorb nonrecyclables can be given on a regular basis and this may control uremia; however, volume control would still be a challenge.

Reference

1. Teschan PE, Ahmad S, Hull AR et al. Panel conference. Daily dialysis—applications and problems. *Trans Am Soc Artif Intern Organs* 1980, 26:600–602.

Index